THE CRAFT

DIY HAIR & Beauty

BY LOU TEASDALE

THE CRAFT by Lou Teasdale

First published in 2014 by Hardie Grant Books

Hardie Grant Books (UK)
Dudley House, North Suite
34–35 Southampton Street
London WC2E 7HF
www.hardiegrant.co.uk

Hardie Grant Books (Australia)
Ground Floor, Building 1
658 Church Street
Melbourne, VIC 3121
www.hardiegrant.com.au

British Library Cataloguing-in-Publication Data. A catalogue record
for this book is available from the British Library.

ISBN: 978-174270-701-3

Publisher: Kate Pollard
Desk Editor: Kajal Mistry
Editor: Rose Gardner
Photography © Masha Mel and Justin Borberly
Photography on page 57 © St Tropez
Images of products from FUDGE, Bond-a-Weave, Halo, BLEACH London, Schwarzkopf,
Bumble & Bumble, Babyliss, Jose Eber, Tangle Teezer, Crown Brushes, MAC, Chantacaille,
Chanel, NIP+FAB, Collection 2000, St Tropez, Barry M, Shimmer Twins, Maybelline, NYX,
Max Factor, Nars, Make Up For Ever, Elf Studio, H&H © the respective brand, used with
thanks from the author. Every attempt has been made to contact the copyright holders. The
publishers would like to hear from any copyright holders who have not been attributed.
Design: Eve Lee
Illustration: Farran Krentcil
Production: Krystal Rodriguez at The Book Agency
Colour Reproduction by p2d

Printed and bound in China by 1010

10 9 8 7 6 5 4 3 2 1

THE CRAFT

DIY HAIR & BEAUTY

BY LOU TEASDALE

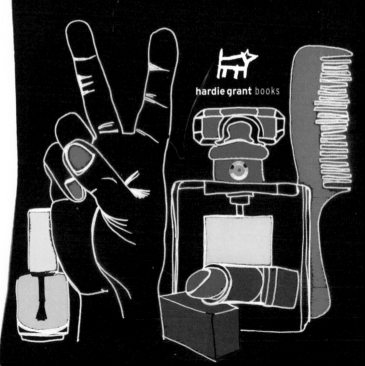

hardie grant books

Contents

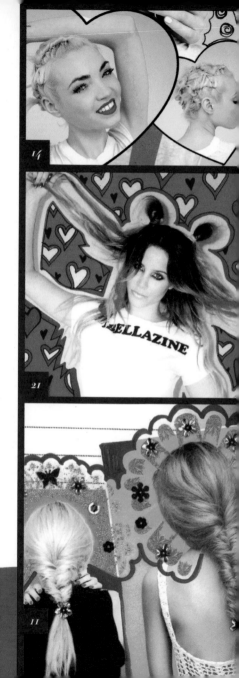

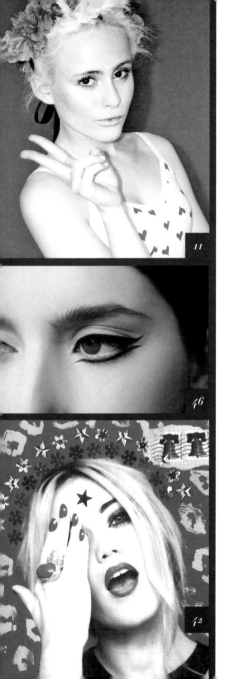

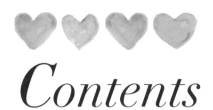

Contents

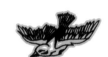

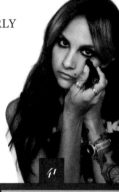

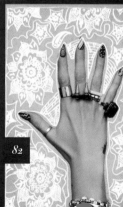

LOU TEASDALE

HAIRDRESSER/MAKE-UP ARTIST/BLOGGER/MUM

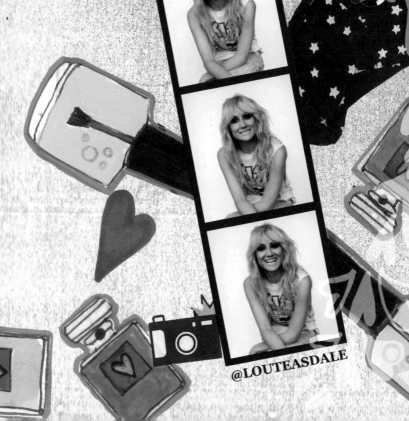

@LOUTEASDALE

WHAT'S YOUR NAME?

Ian teasdale

WHEN IS YOUR BIRTHDAY?

11th October 1983

DRAW YOUR FAVOURITE THING?

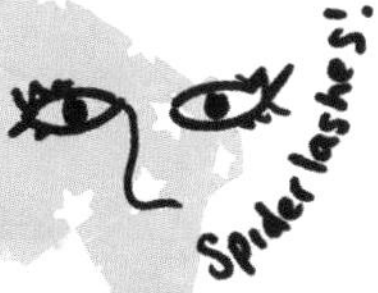

Spider lashes!

WHO ARE YOUR INSPIRATIONS?

Val Garland
Lucy Bridge
Faran Krentzil

WHO'S THE COOLEST PERSON YOU HAVE EVER WORKED WITH?

Juergen Teller

FROM

Yorkshire

LIVES

London

EDUCATION?

London College of FASHION

HOW DOES YOUR CAREER TIMELINE LOOK?

2004 > ASSISTING
↓
'06-'04 > EDITORIAL
↓
'07-'11 > X FACTOR
↓
2011 MUMMY
↓
'11-'14 > PERSONAL SLEB MAKEUP ARTIST
↓
Published Author! ♥

TOP 3 BRANDS?

FUDGE
BUMBLE + bumble
BARRY M

HOW MANY TWITTER FOLLOWERS DO YOU HAVE?

1 MILLION

BEAUTY IS ...

a Religion

7

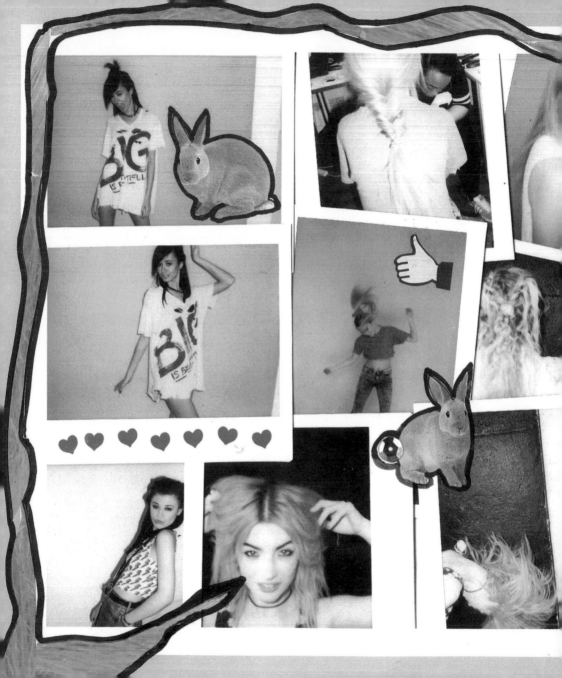

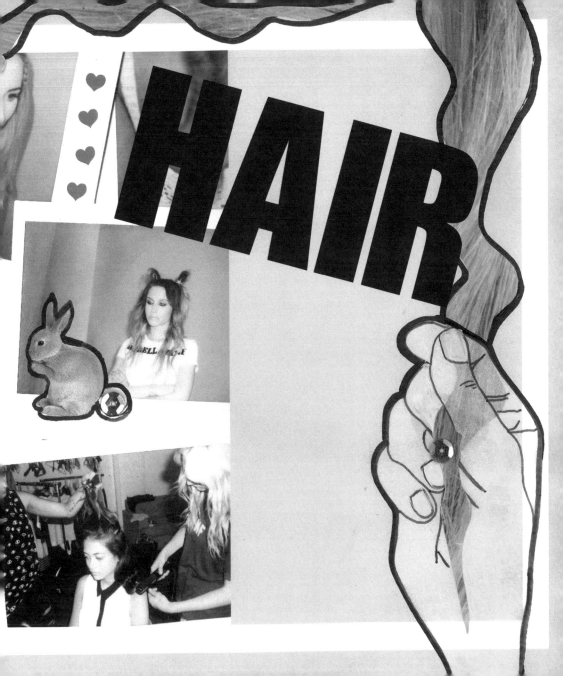

HAIR

BRAINS

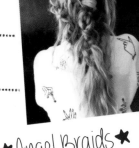

THE FISHTAIL BRAID might look complicated, but it's one of the easiest braids to do.

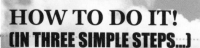

★Angel Braids★

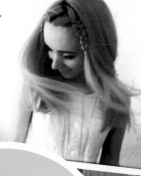

HOW TO DO IT!
(IN THREE SIMPLE STEPS...)

STEP 1.
Split the hair into two big sections, straight down the middle, instead of the three you need for a standard braid.

STEP 2.
Take a thin strand from the outside of the right section and cross it over to join with the left section. Then take a strand from the left section and bring it across to join the right. Repeat until you reach the end.

STEP 3.
Tie the braid off. Then mess it up and tease it apart – be rough! Pull and tug the sides to loosen it up. Braids need to be messy so you don't look like it's your first day of school.

TIP
If your hair is too fine to get the chunky braid you desire then ADD SOME WEAVE to bulk it out!
You can either tie or clip it in. Buy your weave from your local Afro hair shop or order it online (see page 20).

10

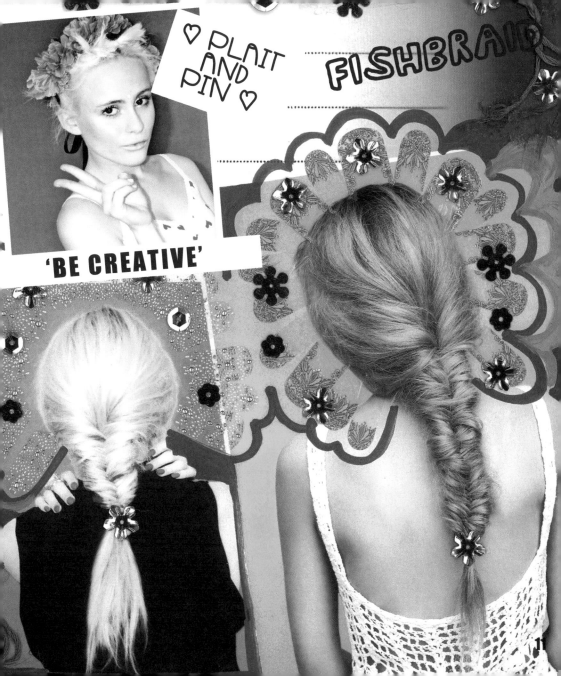

♡ PLAIT AND PIN ♡

FISHBRAID

'BE CREATIVE'

11

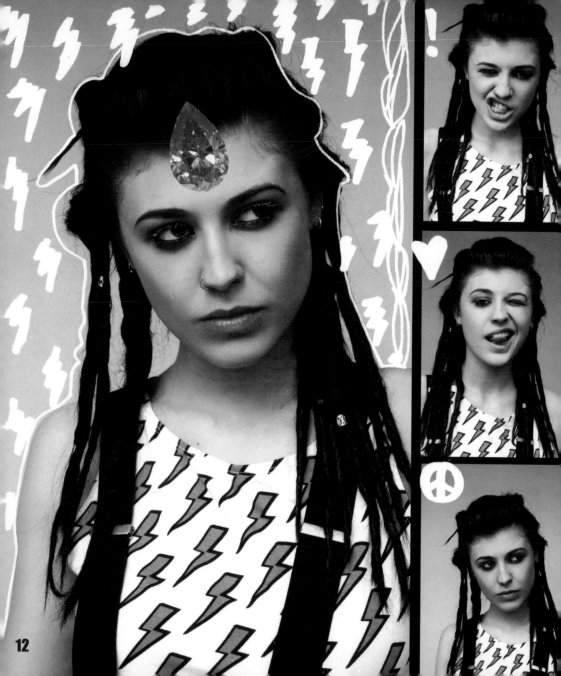

The new DREADLOCK *(it's temporary don't panic!)*

For those of you whose hair is a bit long, straight and boring, here's a good way to jazz it up... NOTE: This is only for girls with hair that's one length – it doesn't really work with layers.

HOW TO DO IT

(NOTE: this takes ages so make sure you've got a good half an hour.)

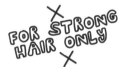

FOR STRONG HAIR ONLY

STEP 1.
Section off and clip the top layers of your hair out of the way.

STEP 2.
Take a small section of hair from the underside. Starting at the top, twist and back-comb it, working your way down to the bottom.

STEP 3.
Spray generously on the top and bottom of the twist with *FUDGE Matte Hed Gas* or anything you have that has a **STRONG HOLD!**

STEP 4.
Keep twisting, back-combing and spraying until it feels like a dreadlock. Repeat steps 1–4 across your whole head.

STEP 5.
Once your whole head is dreadlocked, add hair cuffs and accessories to make it fun :)

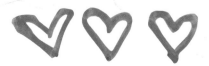

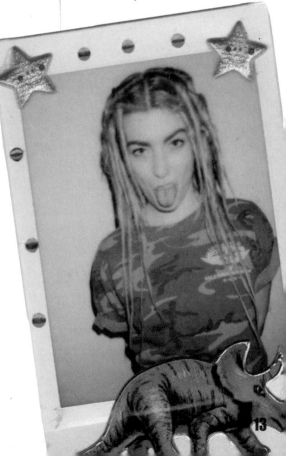

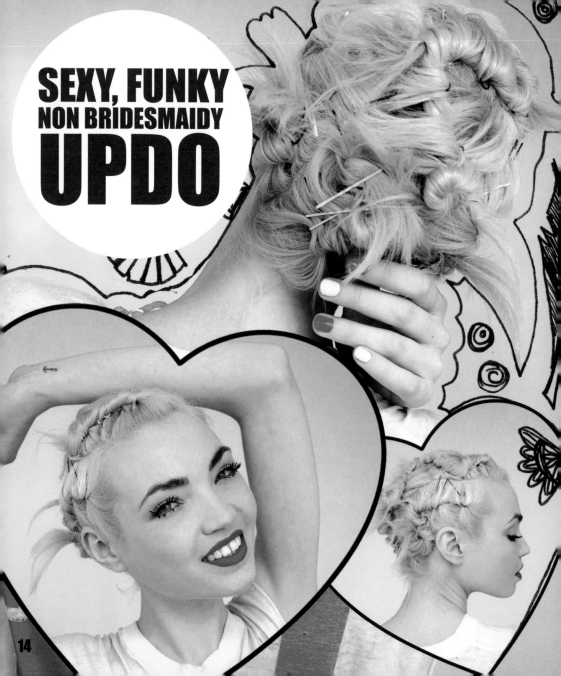

SEXY, FUNKY
NON BRIDESMAIDY
UPDO

If you're attending a wedding and/or wearing a polo neck then reference Björk with this cool updo!

The secret to any successful updo is adding a load of dry shampoo or texture product.

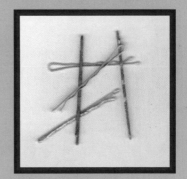

HOW TO DO IT

STEP 1. TO PREP

Add plenty of texture to dry hair, from the roots to the ends. I recommend *FUDGE Urban Powder Styler* or *Batiste Dry Shampoo XXL*. Be careful not to use too much though – it's easy to overdo it.

UPDO TIP: CREATE IT PERFECT THEN MESS IT UP.

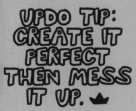

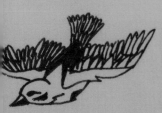

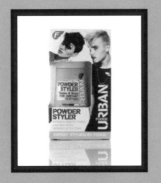

STEP 2. TWIST AND PIN

Take a small section of hair at the front of your head and twist until it coils back on itself. Pin firmly with two crossed grips and blast with *FUDGE Urban Texture Blaster* or a firm hairspray. Build your twists across your head, left to right, pinning sections as you go.

STEP 3. TO FINISH

Once your updo is complete, create splashes of colour with hair chalk! This is a cool temporary way of adding colour to your hair. Here I've used *FUDGE Urban Hair Chalk* in white to give a matte look. There are other products available or you can even use soft art pastels.

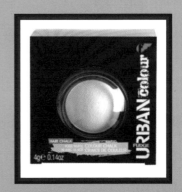

15

TRENDSPOTTING – MULLETS

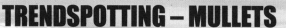

If you have a fringe and fancy shaking things up, try adding extra length to the back with some clip-ins, and give your look a 90s mullet edge.

Don't have a fringe and want one? DO IT YOURSELF! Cut it messy – leave it just that little bit too long and wear it to the side to hide any rough cutting. Invest in a pair of hair scissors and thinning scissors and learn to trim your fringe yourself. This will save on trips to the salon and prevent your bangs being cut way too short by your hairdresser!

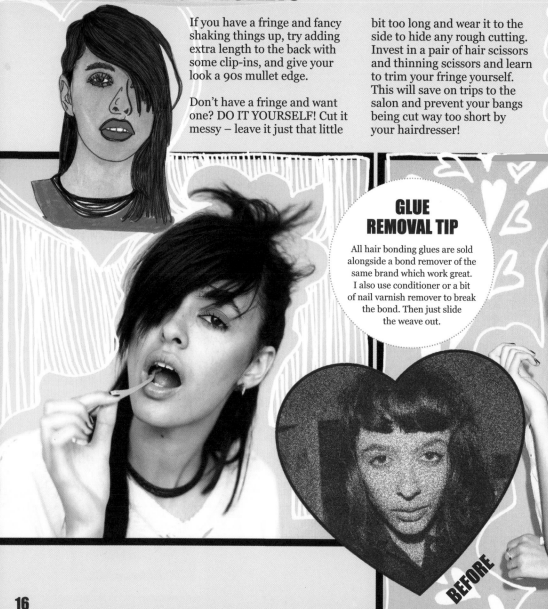

GLUE REMOVAL TIP

All hair bonding glues are sold alongside a bond remover of the same brand which work great. I also use conditioner or a bit of nail varnish remover to break the bond. Then just slide the weave out.

BEFORE

YOU'LL NEED

- **Halo** clip-in hair extensions
- **Bond-A-Weav** liquid gold hair extension glue (optional)
- **FUDGE Matte Hed Gas** or **Bumble & Bumble Surf Spray**
- **Scissors**

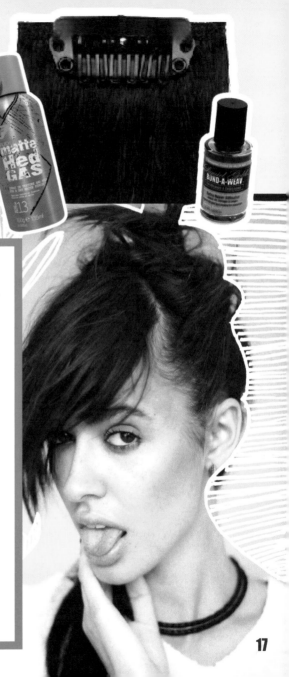

HOW TO DO IT

This look is super-quick to pull off and looks really effective.

STEP 1.
Part your fringe to the side.

STEP 2.
Lift up a layer of your fringe and clip or glue in an extension beneath.

STEP 3.
Add another extension as in Step 2, and repeat with more until you have the desired thickness.

STEP 4.
Grab your scissors and chip away at the extensions, taking care not to cut your own hair. This will make it blend in with your own hair more naturally.

STEP 5.
Blast with your chosen hairspray for hold and texture.

17

PLAT

So you have bleached hair and no matter how white your salon manages to get it, it still goes that gross brassy yellow colour after a while. Don't despair: try a silver shampoo to reclaim the ash.

WE LIKE

FUDGE Paintbox Whiter Shade of Pale

BLEACH London White Toner

Schwarzkopf Professional BC Color Save Silver Shampoo

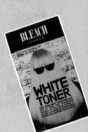

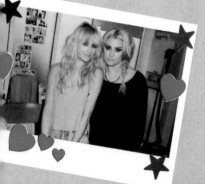

DIY Silver Shampoo
(this is what we do) ...

Buy some granny blue rinse off the Internet, pour a teaspoon amount into a pump spray bottle and add water. Test on a strand of hair. Add more or less dye depending on the effect you want. Once you're happy with the result, direct the spray onto your brassy patches.

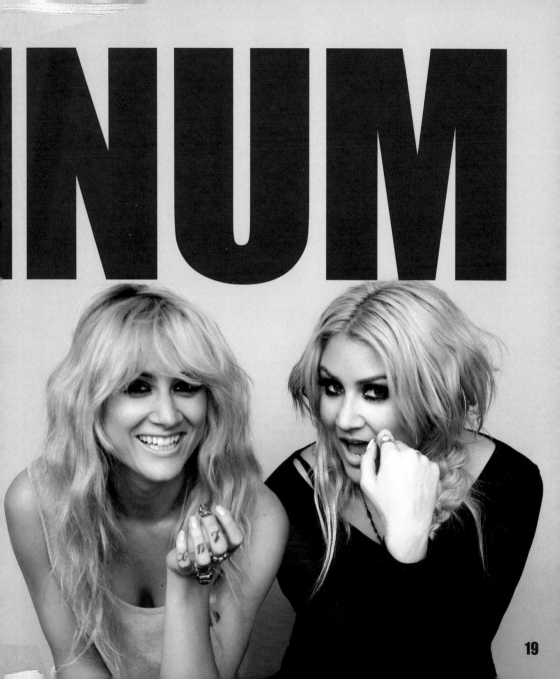

INUM

CLIP-IN CHIC

If you're in the nought-point-two per cent of women who are actually happy with the length and fullness of their hair, you can stop reading now. BYE! The rest of you, HI! I have a really good solution and it doesn't involve hair extensions that cost the world.

Get some **WEAVE**! You can colour it, cut it, glue it in, clip it in, curl it, crimp it, wash it... basically you can do anything you want with it! You can easily find bags of affordable human hair online. Simply cut to your desired length and then just add it where you need it.

All weave comes in packs in a variety of colours and textures, and depending on what you buy you may need to cut it to length. You can buy hair with clips already sewn on or you can sew your own on. You can buy 100% human hair or synthetic (plastic) hair. Synthetic hair is cheaper but you CAN'T apply heat to synthetic hair as it will melt, so no tonging or straightening.

NO DIPPING REQUIRED!

You can even create your own dip-dye look without putting your own precious hair near the bleach.

HOW TO DO IT

Step 1. Buy some weave that matches your hair colour *and* is longer than your own hair.

Step 2. Get yourself a *DIY DIP DYE KIT from Bleach London* and dye the weave strips before glueing them in.

Step 3. Divide your hair into two sections, tying a bun to the top of your head. Clip your hair extensions in along the parting you have made, making sure your own hair falls over the top so they are not visible.

Step 4. You're now ready to hit the streets with style. Our model was back to work with her normal hair on Monday morning – it's that simple!

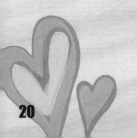

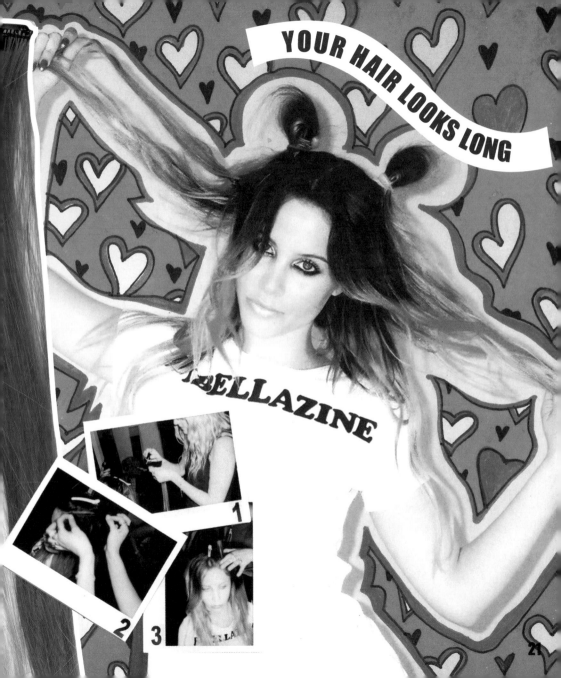

BELLAZINE

1

2

3

RAINBOW HAIR

RAINBOW COLOURS

Look amazing! You'll need blonde or bleached hair to achieve this look. White blondes can get a pastel rainbow effect while golden blondes should opt for darker, brighter tones. Your rainbow can be composed of a variety of vegetable dyes, arranged in different ways.

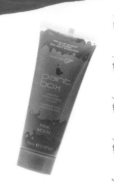

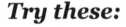

Try these:

CLASSIC
Bright colours! Blend red, orange, yellow, green, blue, indigo and violet, in rainbow order.

STRIPES
Randomly colour sections of hair in different hues. Yellow to pink to blue, and so on.

TWO-TONED
Pick two colours and blend together. If you like red, try matching it with orange, for example.

PASTEL RAINBOW
Apply as per the Classic Rainbow but use softer tones of each colour like candy pink, powder blue and mint green.

GOLDFINGER

CHILLI

RED CORVETTE

CHERRY BOMB

VENDETTA RED

RASBERRY BERET

BLUEBERRY HILL

PURPLE HAZE

BLUE VELVET

BLUE HAWAII

PINK MOON

PRETTY FLAMINGO

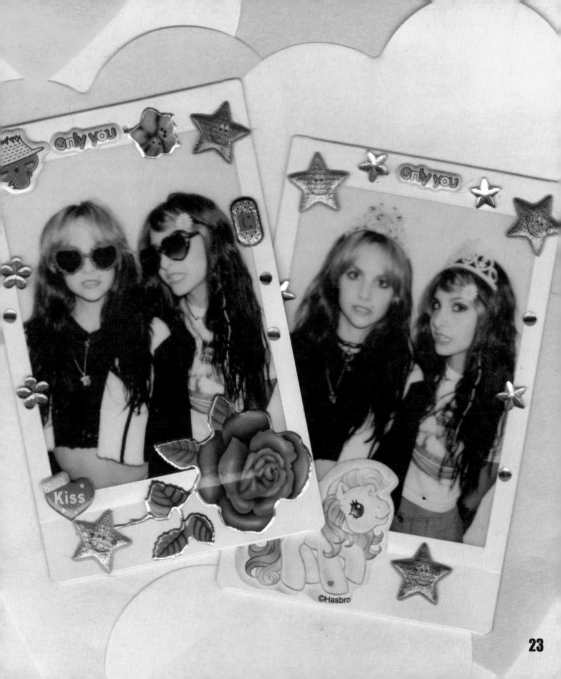

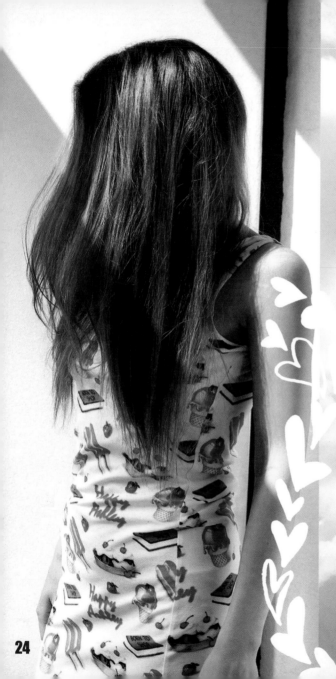

RAINBOW RECIPES

Get the right colour for you. We call them **RECIPES** because it's like cooking! Add conditioner to your mix to 'water down' the colour and make it paler. The less conditioner, the bolder the colour. Once you have applied the colour it's up to you how long you leave it on — the longer you leave it the stronger the colour. Always shampoo your hair and apply **CRAZY COLOUR** to damp hair.

Rainbow Recipes

1/2 PINK MOON
+1/2 WHITER SHADE OF PALE
= PINKERTON

PINK MOON BY FUDGE

1/4 TURQUOISE BLUE
+ 3/4 WHITER SHADE OF PALE
= GREENDAY

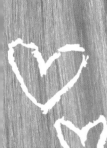

1/2 BLUEBERRY HILL
+ 1/2 TURQUISE BLUE
= PURPLE HAZE

DRAINBOW

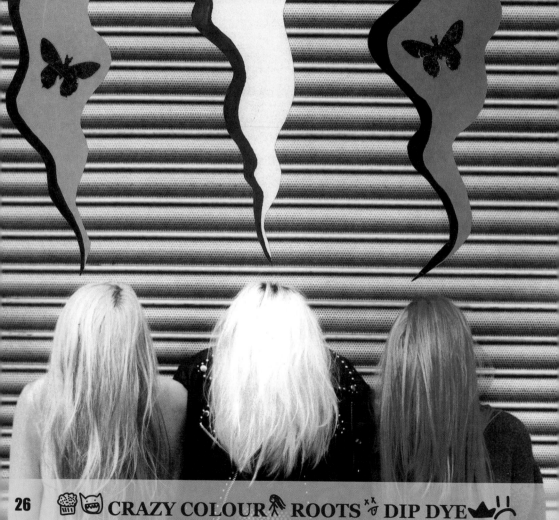

CRAZY COLOUR ROOTS DIP DYE

DRAINBOW — WASHED-OUT RAINBOW HAIR

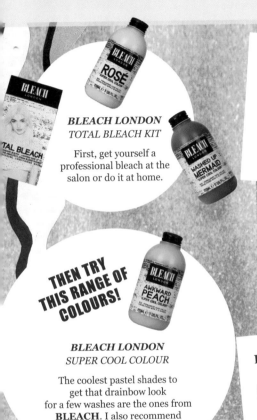

BLEACH LONDON
TOTAL BLEACH KIT

First, get yourself a professional bleach at the salon or do it at home.

THEN TRY THIS RANGE OF COLOURS!

BLEACH LONDON
SUPER COOL COLOUR

The coolest pastel shades to get that drainbow look for a few washes are the ones from **BLEACH**. I also recommend *Directions in 'Lilac'* as a cool shade to use.

Those cool people who live in East London were first on the scene with neon/lumo/vunge green/pink hair last year. And when the dye started to wash out, they accidentally created a whole new look: drainbow! It's a much more WEARABLE COLOUR trend that's great for girls who don't want to go too crazy with their pretty hair!

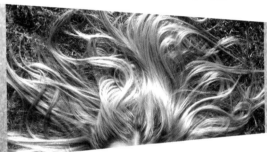

HOW TO DO IT

Step 1. You'll need naturally pale or bleached hair as a base for colour. If you're going lighter, get it done at a salon or use a professional bleaching kit like the one from **BLEACH LONDON**.

Step 2. Buy yourself some crazy coloured hair dye in pink/purple/blue/green/whatever you fancy, and simply mix in a little with your conditioner.

Step 3. You'll only notice a subtle difference on the first go but colour will build over subsequent washes to give you Kate Moss candyfloss hair!

GRUNGE HAIR

To create **GRUNGE HAIR** it is all about selecting the right hair product for your hair texture!

HOW TO DO IT

STEP 1.

Bring out the natural wave in your hair, even if your hair is straight. Do this by applying a texture spray (salt spray) or a thickening spray, then twist your hair into curls using your fingers. If you have one, use a diffuser hairdryer to scrunch it dry. Flip from hot to cold hair at medium pressure so your hair doesn't get frizzy!

STEP 2.

Once dry your hair may need defining or smoothing. Using your hair straighteners, take large sections of your hair and push into an 'S' shape, pressing the straighteners on top. This will create a flattering, natural wave.

STEP 3:

If your hair is dry, finish off with a bit of oil/serum through your mid-lengths and ends. For hair that feels too clean, use brilliantine like ***Bumble & Bumble*** or a matte styling cream – I use ***FUDGE Matte Hed Gas.*** This adds separation / grit so your hair feels slept-in and grungy!

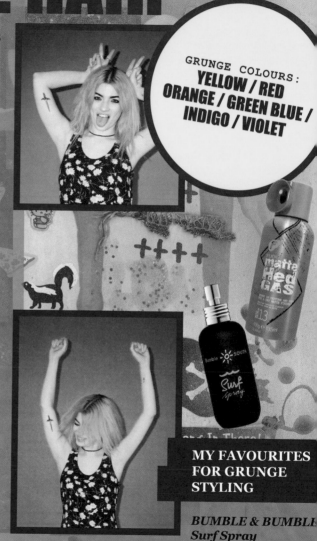

GRUNGE COLOURS:
YELLOW / RED ORANGE / GREEN BLUE / INDIGO / VIOLET

MY FAVOURITES FOR GRUNGE STYLING

BUMBLE & BUMBLE Surf Spray

FUDGE Matte Hed Gas

28

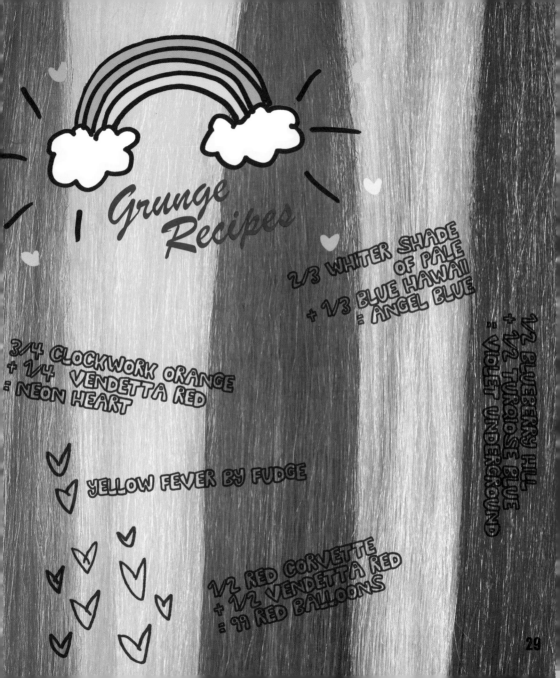

Grunge Recipes

2/3 WHITER SHADE
OF PALE
+ 1/3 BLUE HAWAII
= ANGEL BLUE

3/4 CLOCKWORK ORANGE
+ 1/4 VENDETTA RED
= NEON HEART

YELLOW FEVER BY FUDGE

1/2 BLUEBERRY HILL
+ 1/2 TURQUOSE BLUE
= VIOLET UNDERGROUND

1/2 RED CORVETTE
+ 1/2 VENDETTA RED
= 99 RED BALLOONS

ACCESSORIES

Sometimes less is more. Then again, sometimes it's not! I think you should just go for it with hair accessories. Just when you think you've added enough, keep going! Be creative when sourcing your bobbles, clips, beads and slides. Children's toy shops have some great trinkets and all kids' clothes shops have good accessories sections too. Look on eBay. Go to markets and check small supermarkets. Vintage costume jewellery shops are also good for hair slides.

Scrunchies are back and all over the shops. For an effortless Clueless look go for a scrunchie topknot!

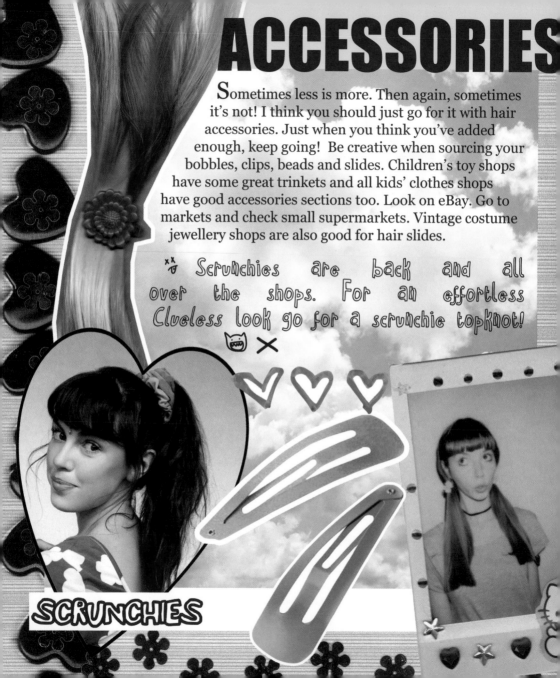

SCRUNCHIES

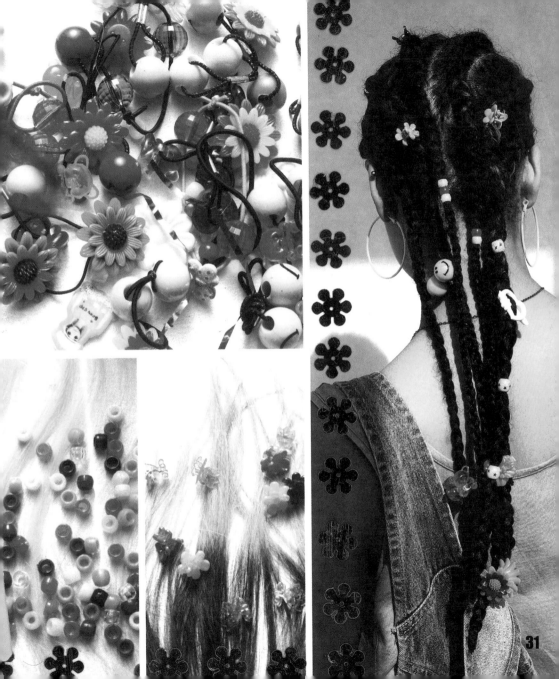

31

ESSENTIAL HAIR TOOLS

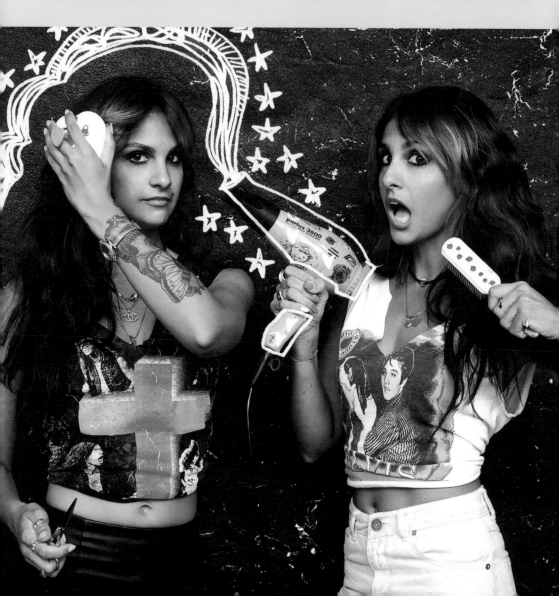

THINNERS

Thinning scissors are an absolute necessity if you're gonna get creative with your hair. These are perfect for blending a new fringe, shortening your weave or feathering your ends for grungy hair. You can pick these up at a chemist or online.

TANGLE TEEZER

If you haven't tried this detangling marvel, get one in your life.

BIG HAIR by BABYLISS

If you like a froofy blow-dry from the salon but struggle to achieve it then this is brilliant. It actually gives you a salon blow-dry at home.

JOSÉ EBER TONG

These come in three sizes. The large iron is the best for loose curls. It gets super hot, which is the key to a curl that holds. These irons aren't cheap but they create great a tousled look. Simply rough dry your hair then loosely wrap chunks and ends around the iron – and away you go!

LARGE ROUND VENT BRUSH

Once you've finished your hairstyle, whether it be straight or loosely curled, quickly blow-dry your front sections or fringe around one of these to give a more 'finished' look.

DEEP WAVER by BABYLISS

This is THE BEST tool for getting beachy, wavy, cool hair – I use it every single day! It's totally unique and no other product can give you a wave like this. An absolute must-have for me!

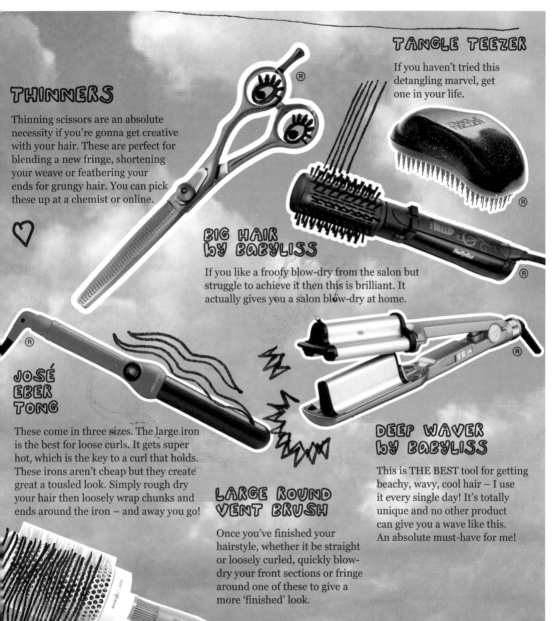

33

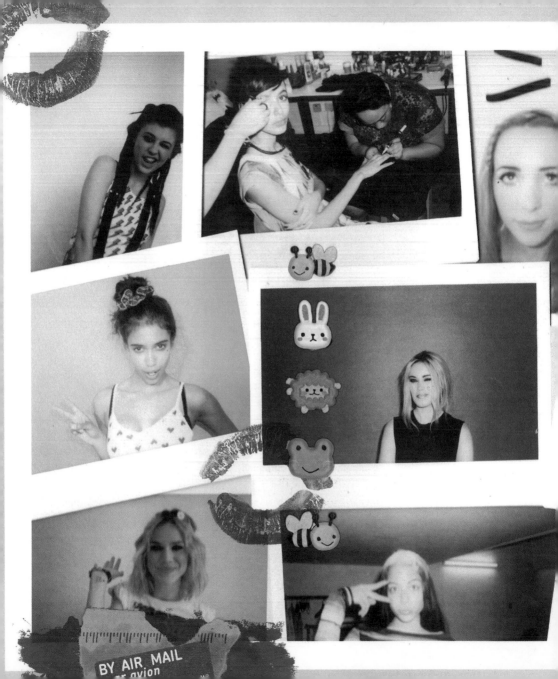

MAKE-UP

SUPERBASE

A good tinted moisturiser is the key to my favourite make-up look
– the make-up that makes the world go round, the make-up
everyone needs to learn how to achieve. Which is . . .
NO MAKE-UP MAKE-UP! ❦

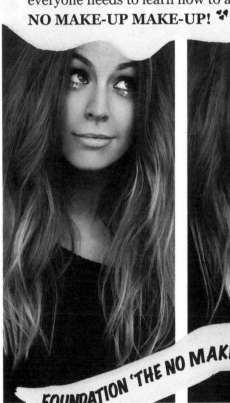
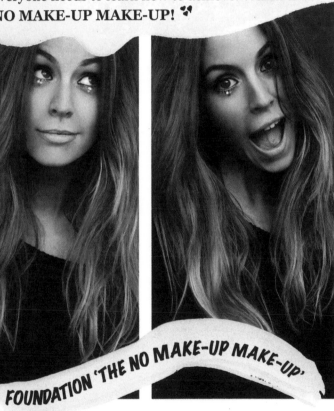
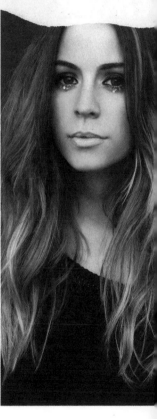

FOUNDATION 'THE NO MAKE-UP MAKE-UP'

TIP! THE KEY TO THIS LOOK IS FINDING YOUR PERFECT BASE.
GET TESTERS. ASK FOR SKIN MAKEOVERS AT BEAUTY COUNTERS.
DON'T STOP UNTIL YOU FIND THE PERFECT PRODUCT! I LOVE . . .

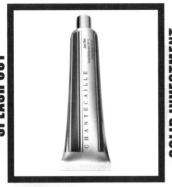

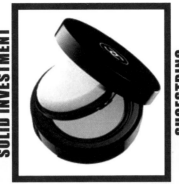

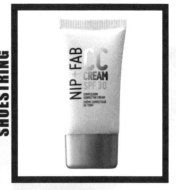

CHANTECAILLE
TINTED MOISTURISER

It's pretty expensive, but this really is the perfect foundation. It's the only tinted moisturiser I've ever used that doesn't require you to apply a base moisturiser beforehand. It also has really good coverage. So if you're loaded, ~~lend us a tenner~~ then splash out on this!

CHANEL
TEINT INNOCENCE CREME

I use this foundation loads. It's has really good coverage yet is still sheer. It may be Chanel but here's a hot tip: if you just buy refills, it's actually a really good price!

NIP+FAB
CC CREAM

This tinted moisturiser is fantastic for everyday wear. You may need to use a bit more concealer if you have blemishes or dark circles, but it's great for evening-out the skin tone – and it's super cheap!

C436 Mini Duo Fibre Blender by Crown Brush

'No make-up' make-up isn't about not wearing any make-up. Once you've perfected your base, you'll need some colour. But rather than covering your cheeks with bronzer or blusher, try using a loose bronzer or tan pigment combined with a **mixing medium**. Mixing medium will change your life! It's a liquid that you add to make-up to concoct your own special potions. It makes colours more vivid and helps make-up stay put (so it's great to add to eye-shadows too). Find some at a good cosmetics store or online.

Mix some of your tinted moisturiser and tan pigment or bronzer with the mixing medium until you have a perfect sunkissed shade, then apply with a good brush (like the one above from **Crown**) around the outside of your face to create a very subtle glowing tan. If you like rosy cheeks, try mixing some pink instead of bronze and apply to the apples of your cheeks. Remember, the desired effect is natural so don't overdo it and **blend, blend, blend!**

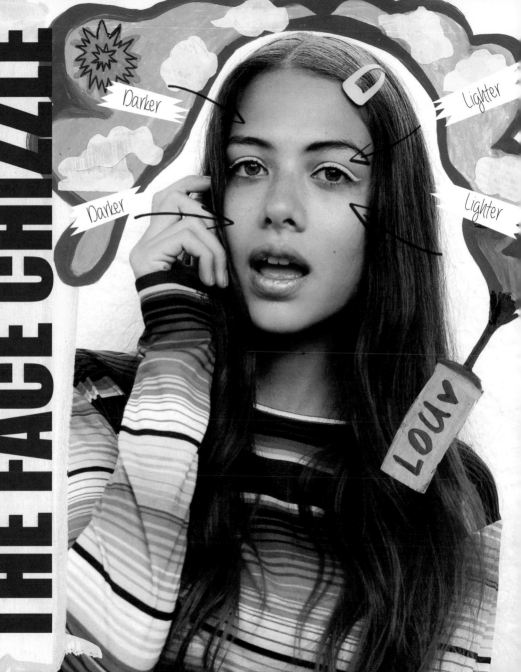

CONTOURING IS SIMPLE...

Contouring is a make-up technique that uses light and shade to shape and highlight parts of your face.

Here's how!

Look at your face in a mirror and see where the light naturally highlights it – along your cheekbones, the bridge of your nose and the bow of your lip. Sweep light-reflective products with a shimmer over these areas.

Then apply bronzer or a special contour powder (available from good beauty stores) to the darker areas of your face: along the hairline, jawline and under your cheekbones. Blend well!

MY FAVOURITE CONTOUR PRODUCTS!
(For all budgets)

SHOESTRING

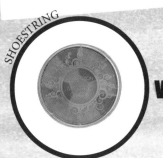

VS

SOLID INVESTMENT

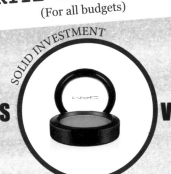

VS

SPLASH OUT

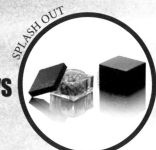

Collection 2000
Shimmering Mosiac Glow

Super-cheap and a great colour, this powder has a pink undertone that combats 'orange face' and a really nice shimmer for an evening look.

MAC
'Taupe Shape' by Mac

This a solid investment and a is great matte option for day contouring.

St Tropez
Bronzing Rocks

Expensive, but worth it. Wear it in the day, in the evening – whenever. It's the best bronzer in the world!

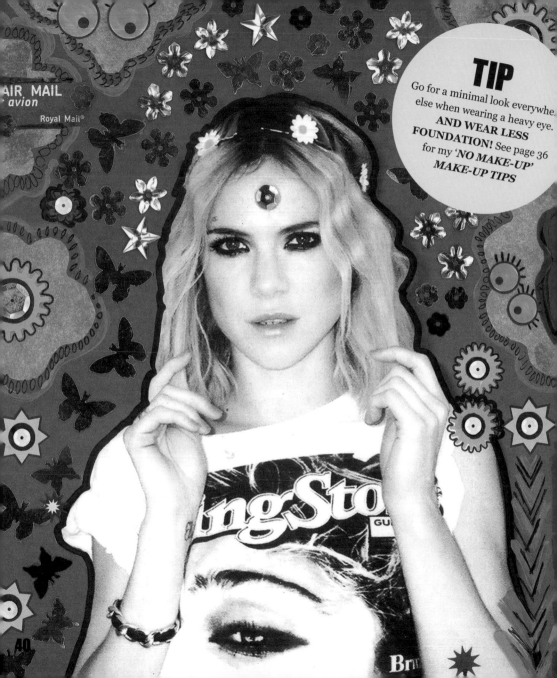

AIR MAIL
par avion

Royal Mail®

TIP

Go for a minimal look everywhe.
else when wearing a heavy eye.
**AND WEAR LESS
FOUNDATION!** See page 36
for my *'NO MAKE-UP'*
MAKE-UP TIPS

40

SMOKY
SMUDGEY
GREASY
EYE

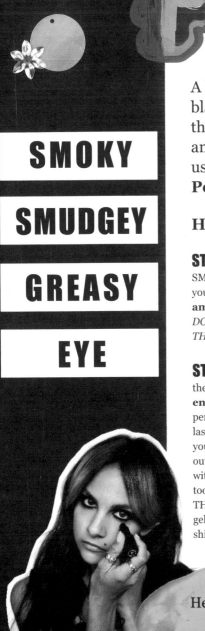

A little pot of **MAC Liquid Fluidline** in black is the key product for this look. And the tools to create it are simply **your finger** and a **Kohl eyeliner**. My fave eyeliner to use for this is **Barry M Black Kohl Pencil** – and it's cheap!

HOW TO DO IT

STEP 1. Using your finger, SMUDGE the liquid gel around your eye, just up to the crease. **Be ambitious** if you like but *PLEASE DON'T GO ANYWHERE NEAR THE BROW!*

STEP 2. DUNK your eyeliner into the gel. **Eyeliner just isn't black enough without a dunk.** Just pencil around your eye as close to the lashes as possible, then pencil inside your upper and lower lids, and flick out at the corners. This works nicely with any other coloured eyeshadow too! Apply your eyeshadow as normal THEN just dip your eyeliner in the gel and frame the eye with a bit of shiny blackness.

★ CHEAT

Heres a quick fix for this look. Get yourself a black lipstick and *SMUDGE* away!

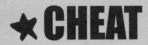

A MODERN LIP

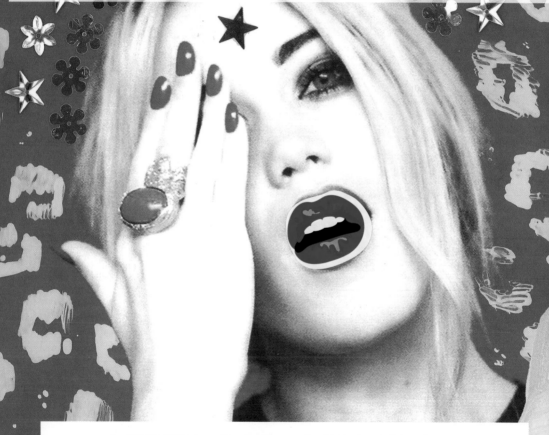

(JUST ADD POWDER)

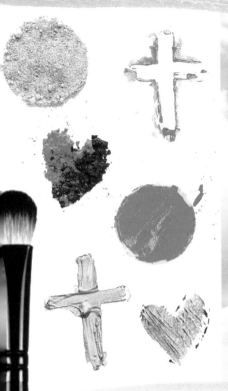

MATTE LIPS

Colours are going to get colder, but make sure you don't end up looking dodgy with this latest beauty trend. I would opt for *Barry M lipstick in 'Lilac'* and *MAC 'Pink Opal'* pigment on top for a softer version.

Shu Uemura Beige Lipstick is great but very matte, so prep your lips with a lip balm before use so they don't dry out. After you've applied it, blot well. If you load on too much, you'll end up suffering. from 'nude-liporexia'.

LOWERING THE TONE
Why not try a red lip with orange powder on top to mix it up?

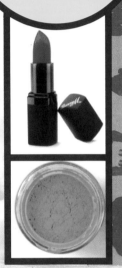

HOW TO DO IT!
Once you've selected the colour there are THREE SIMPLE STEPS to remember!

STEP 1.
Prep your lips with lip balm before adding matte layers to avoid them looking dry and REMEMBER TO STICK THE BALM IN YOUR BAG FOR LATER ON!

STEP 2.
Apply a good layer of your chosen lip colour.

STEP 3.
Using your finger or a flat eyeshadow brush, press a matching eyeshadow on top of your lipstick. All done!

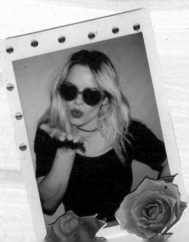

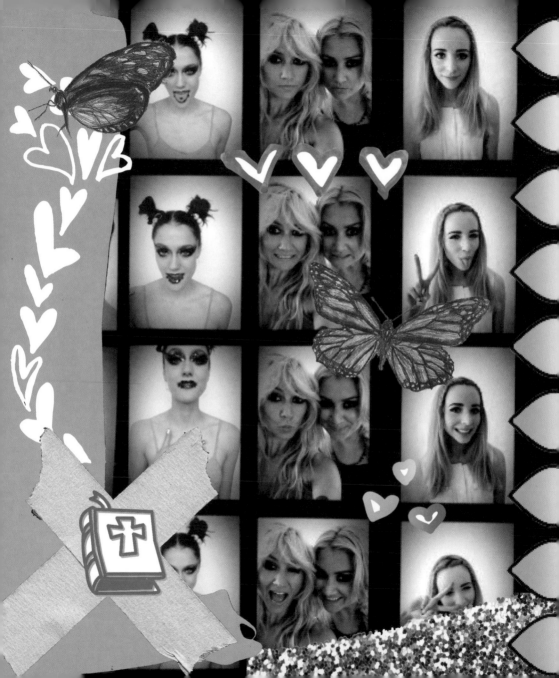

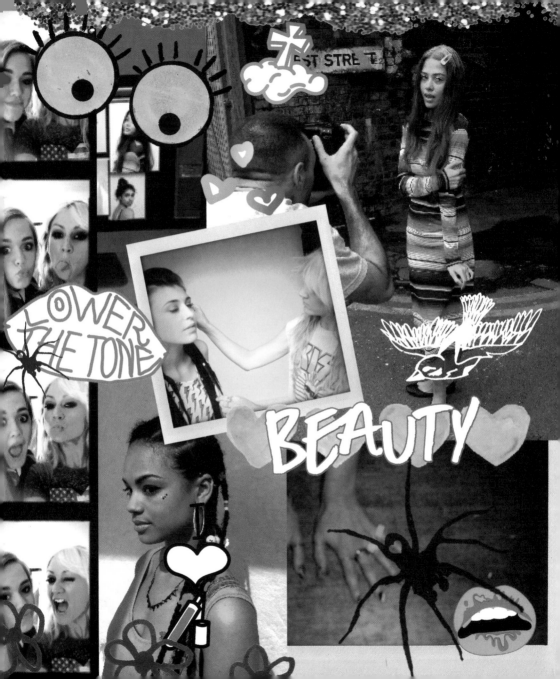

LOWER THE TONE

BEAUTY

EYELINER

BOBBI BROWN eyeliner is the industry favourite for this look, but I've tried some others to give you options. The competitors are...

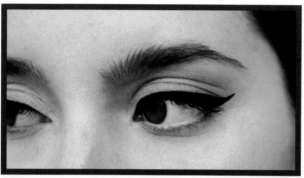

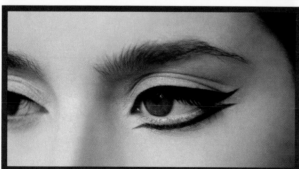

BOBBI BROWN
LONG-WEAR
GEL EYELINER

VS

ESTÉE LAUDER
GEL EYELINER
–
MAC COSMETICS
FLUIDLINE
–
STILA
SMUDGEPOTS

VERDICT

The only contender is *ESTÉE LAUDER GEL EYELINER.* It's a little more expensive than **Bobbi Brown** but you get more and it comes with a little brush!

TIP!

If you're not confident, map your desired flick out with brown eye shadow and then fill it in with eyeliner!

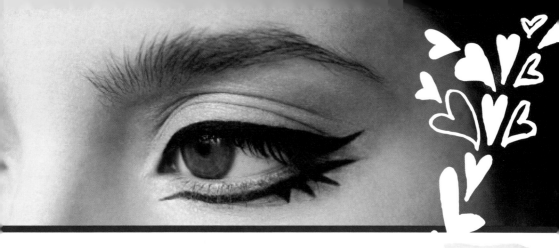

HOW TO APPLY LIQUID LINER

STEP 1.
Prepare your eyelids with primer, or wipe clean with a wet wipe. If you plan on wearing eye shadow, apply it now and your eyeliner will go over the top.

STEP 2.
Using a smooth, swift action, apply your eyeliner on the rim of your eyelid. Lean your elbows on a table to help keep your hand steady.

STEP 3.
For a funky, fun look, flick out the ends, extending the overall shape of your eyes. To really make your eyes pop, apply a line just below your bottom lashes, as above.

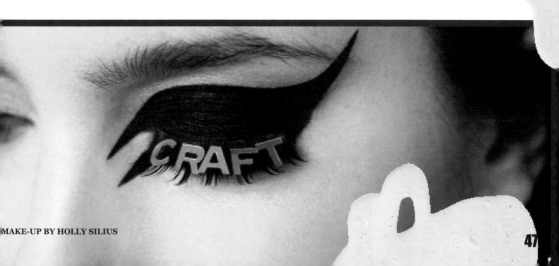

MAKE-UP BY HOLLY SILIUS

NON-TRANNY LASHES

HOLLY

FALSE EYELASHES DON'T HAVE TO LOOK TACKY IF YOU WEAR THEM RIGHT!

Shimmer Twins Lashes are dead fashionable and really cool.

The **Shimmer Twins Treasure Lashes** were created by make-up artist Holly Silius in Dalston in Summer 2011. We spoke to Holly about how she built a successful business from fancy eyelashes!

'These began when I made some peacock feather lashes for a "lash birthday party", then a week later I made a set of lashes that ended up on the cover of _i-D Magazine_ with US rapper KREAYSHAWN. I was then inundated with request for bespoke lashes from friends, drag queens and dancers, so I ended up making a full range of nine designs which are all adorned with glitter, stars, hearts and sequins. They went into ASOS and Urban Outfitters, among other stores, and have been hugely popluar. I still make bespoke ones for special requests, adorned with words and sayings like the "CRAFT" ones I made especially for Lou!'

www.shimmertwins.com

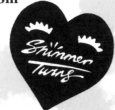

HOW TO APPLY FAKE LASHES

STEP 1.
Take your eyelashes out of the box, hold them against your eyelid and cut them to the width of your lid.

STEP 2.
Squeeze some eyelash glue along the edge of the false lash, being careful not to add too much.

STEP 3.
Allow the glue to dry for longer than you think, depending on how much you have used – it needs to be almost dry. I often do my eyebrows while waiting

STEP 4.
Add the false lash as close to your natural lash as possible, and press into place using a cotton bud.

STEP 5.
Allow the glue to dry for a few minutes before applying your mascara.

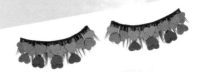

49

BROWSCARA

All the cool kids are doing browscara. What does it remind me of...? Oh wait, remember hair mascara? *THAT*. Even if you're mega blonde you'll still look **COOLER WITH DARK EYEBROWS**. Trust me. You don't even need to faff around with dye. Once you've done your lashes, simply brush some mascara into your brows and **DONE. COOL!**

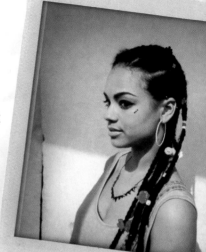

YOU'LL NEED
- *NYX Eyeshadow in Lilac*
- *C216 Stiff Brow Brush from Crown Brush*
- *Maybelline Volum' Express in Colorshock Purple*

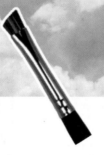
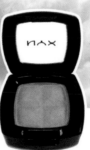

HOW TO DO IT PROPERLY:

Step 1. Use a brightly coloured eye shadow to fill in your brows. extend them slightly with the colour you're using.

Step 2. Use a coloured mascara in a darker tone to brush through your brow hairs. We've used pink on our model. Sounds mad but looks very cool!

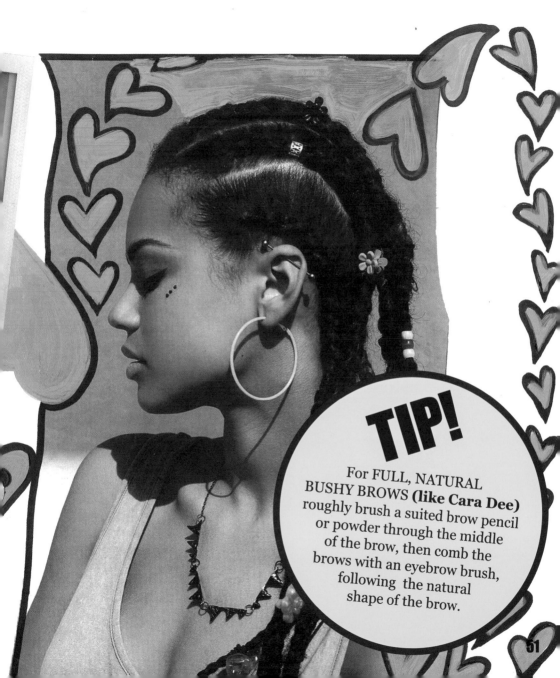

TIP!

For FULL, NATURAL BUSHY BROWS **(like Cara Dee)** roughly brush a suited brow pencil or powder through the middle of the brow, then comb the brows with an eyebrow brush, following the natural shape of the brow.

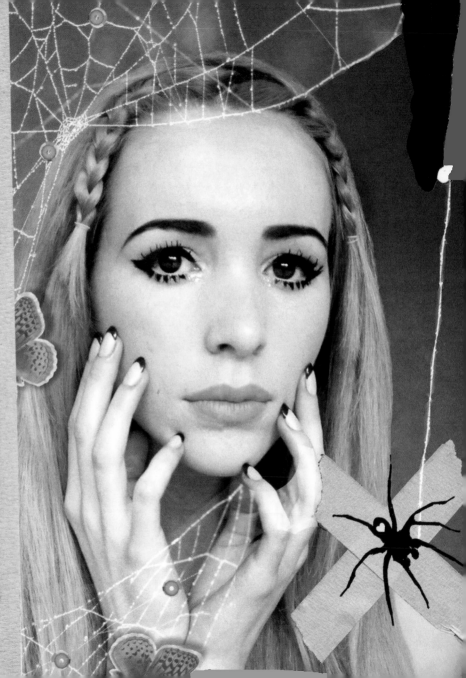

SPIDER LASHES

Forget limp daddy-long-legs lashes.
We're layering our mascara on TEN TIMES.
COS WE WANT TARANTULA LEGS! You don't need
false lashes for this look, just **CLUMP** it up and **LUMP** it on.

~

TRY MAX FACTOR 2000 CALORIE MASCARA
*IT'S PROBABLY THE BEST PRODUCT IN
THE WHOLE WORLD, EVER. EVER!*

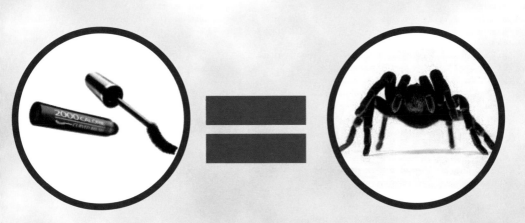

STEP 1. Apply thick layer to your first lash and then to the other lash.

STEP 2. Apply another layer to your first lash again, and then your other lash, again.

STEP 3. Apply another layer to your first lash again, and then your other lash, again.

STEP 4. Apply another layer to your first lash again, and then your other lash, again.

STEP 5. Apply another layer to your first lash again, and then your other lash, again.

STEP 6. Apply another layer to your first lash again, and then your other lash, again.

STEP 7. Once you have applied enough layers, use the pointy tip of your mascara wand to create the spiders legs. You need to clump them together to become triangle-type shapes.

STEP 8. Apply another layer to your first lash again, and then your other lash, again.

TIP! DON'T FORGET YOUR BOTTOM LASHES!!

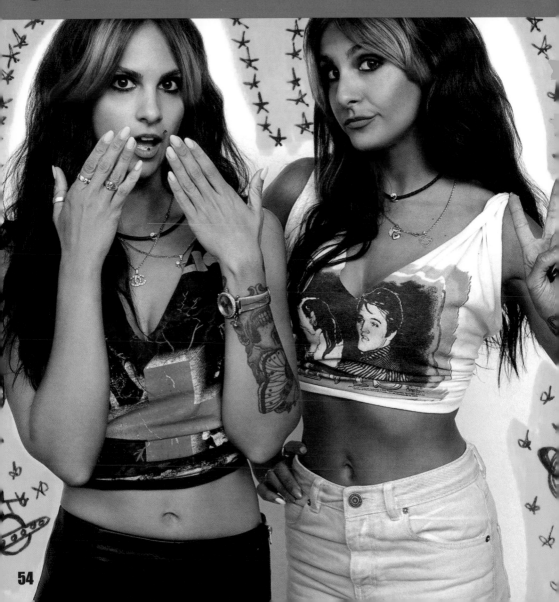

I live in the UK where the weather is significantly colder than those of you who are lucky enough to live in places like LA and Sydney... this makes us the masters of faking a tan. Being a bronzed natural beauty is one of my favourite looks. Applying a light mist of *St Tropez Instant Tan Lotion* to your face can lessen the amount of make-up you need to apply by at least half. *Nars Laguna* is the make-up artists fave – it's the best shade of bronzer I have ever come across – a perfect, non-orange shade without an Oompa Loompa in sight, even on those days where you may need a little extra! However, it's not exactly cheap. I feel it my duty to offer you a bargain alternative. Look out for *Collection 2000 Shimmering Mosaic Glow*. As a make-up artist, I wouldn't use it for a professional job as it's a tiny bit too shiny, but it's a really good pinky tan (the pink tone knocks out the orange and looks more natural like a real suntan) and is great for everyday wear. Best of all, you can buy it with your loose change!

HOW TO BE A BRONZED BABE IN THE SUN

STEP 1.
Apply fake tan to your moisturised face.

STEP 2.
Put more fake tan on (more than that!).

STEP 3.
If you're turning orange then stop. But if you can take it, put bit more on your cheeks and forehead!

STEP 4.
Apply waterproof mascara. We like **BADGal from Benefit** because it's clumpy and doesn't run.

STEP 5.
Apply more mascara. Don't be shy, keep adding more.

STEP 6.
LEAVE YOUR FACE NOW. THAT IS ALL! If you are all hot and bothered, you'll look really gross with extras like foundation, powder, eye roll and blusher. Just leave it, you look nice.

STEP 7.
Leave your hair to do what it does: it's sunny, you're sweating, it's one of those days when you can just leave it.

HOW TO FAKE TAN PROPERLY

TIPS FROM CELEBRITY TANNING EXPERT
JULES HEPTONSTALL

I work with a number of Hollywood A-List celebrities and know the importance of a good, NATURAL-LOOKING fake tan. Here are some pointers to minimising those 'tell-tale' signs – fear not my friends, I'm here to help you!

Step 1. Prep like you've never prepped before: EXFOLIATING is key here. The day before you apply your tan, give your body a good scrub. This will ensure your final colour is uniform, and will also help your tan to fade evenly (scaly tans are not a good look, right?).

Step 2. Use an aloe vera-based moisturiser on your hands, elbows, knees and feet just before you apply your tan. This will ensure that these areas don't go too dark.

Step 3. ALWAYS, always apply your tan with an applicator mitt. Put the tan onto the mitt first and then rub it in to your skin, being careful not to miss any areas.

Step 4. Use what's left on your mitt from your body application for your hands and feet. Don't use a fresh pump of tan on your mitt for these very absorbent areas. It's too much!

Step 5. Wipe your palms and nails after application.

Step 6. Moisturise your body every day with the same aloe vera-based moisturiser as used before in Step 2. This will not only lock in your tan's colour, it will keep your skin soft and hydrated.

Step 7. Never forget – practice makes perfect, and the best fake tan is the one that looks real.

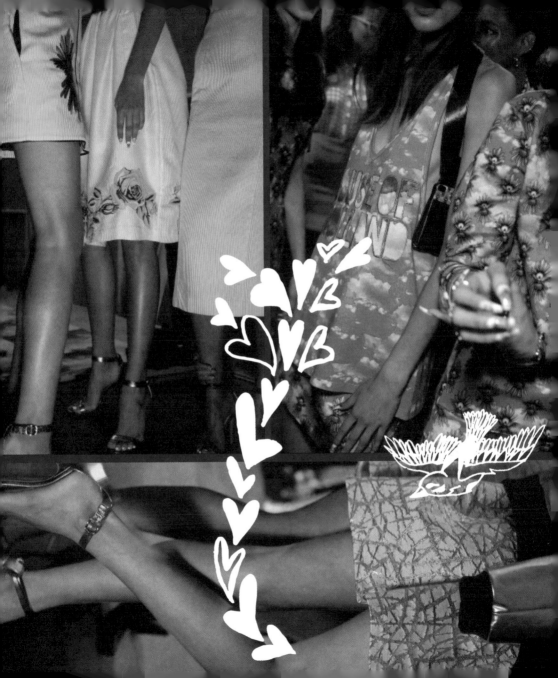

COLOURED MASCARA

You don't need any other make-up for a festival than a coloured mascara. The key is ... LAYERS (see Spider Lashes on page 53). Keep applying until the colour is thick and vibrant and you can't go wrong!

MY FAVOURITES

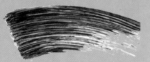

MAYBELLINE

MAKE UP FOR EVER

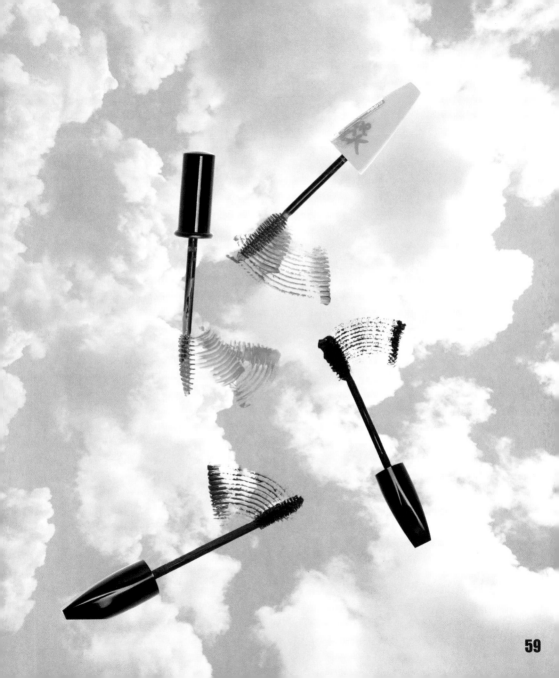

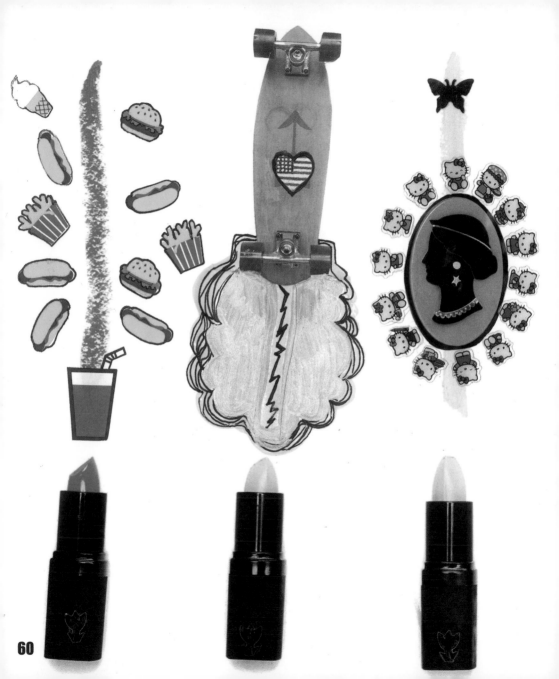

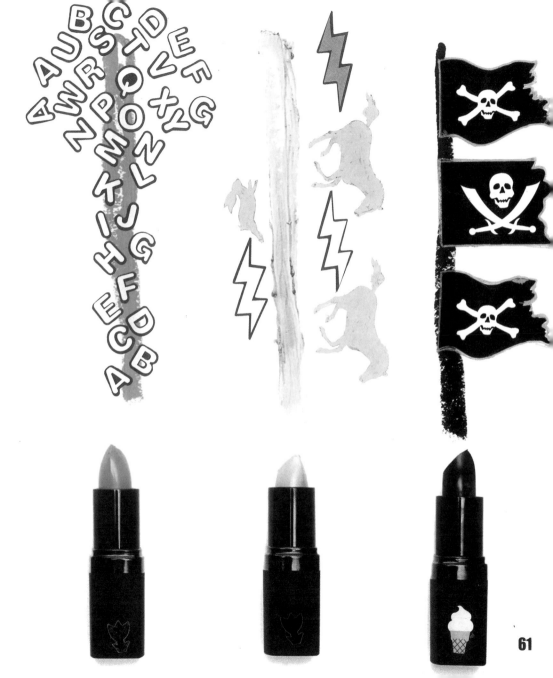

61

A DECORATED FACE

DAYTIME FACE DECOR

Whether you're going to a festival, a garden party, or just hanging out in East London, there are loads of chilled-out looks you can create without looking like you're wearing leftover make-up from a 70s disco the night before. Why not try a simple heart-shaped beauty spot with your eyeliner? Or a small star? It's a super cute touch that gives you edge without crazy colour.

In your entire life of experi*MENTAL* make-up this is probably the most *MENTAL* you're gonna get. So:

1. Choose a texture.

2. Choose a colour

3. Stick to it.

4. Think about where on your face you want to decorate. You can try using glitter as eyeshadow. Or you can use glitter as a high-lighter and apply to the top of your cheekbones and corners of your eye. Or a simple bindi diamanté does the trick!

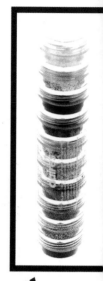

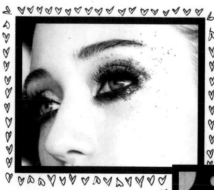

TRY

* *Claire's Accessories* Glitter Stack

* *Suruchi* bindis

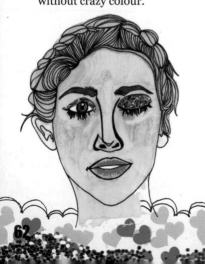

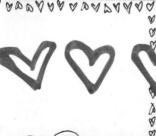

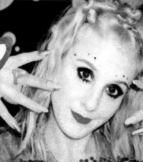

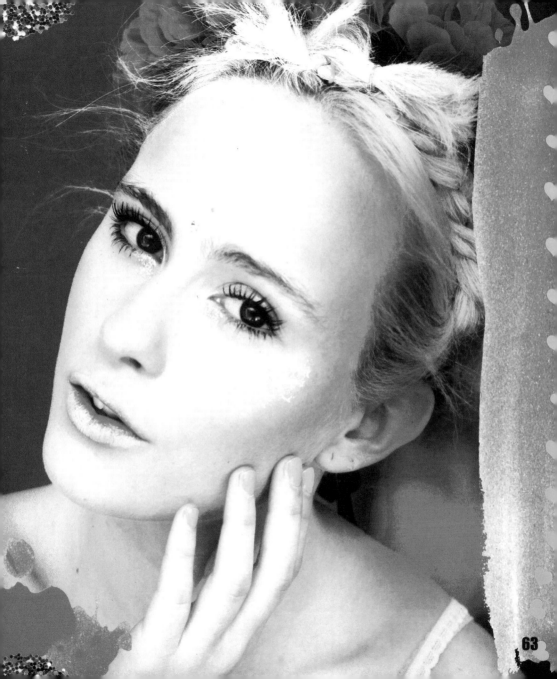

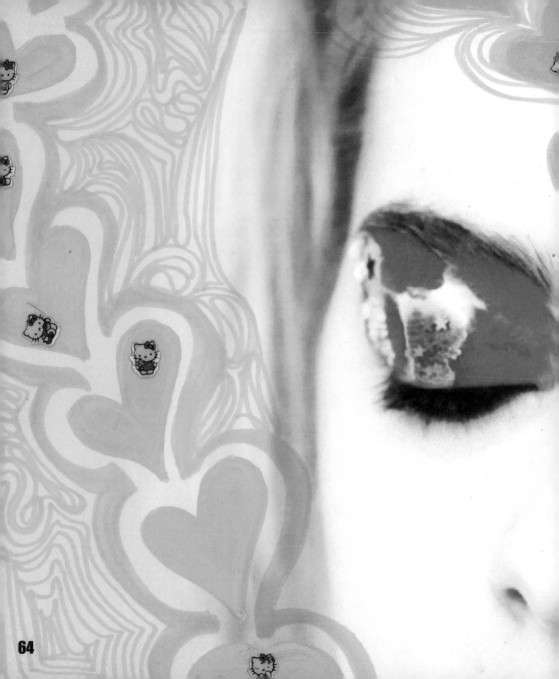

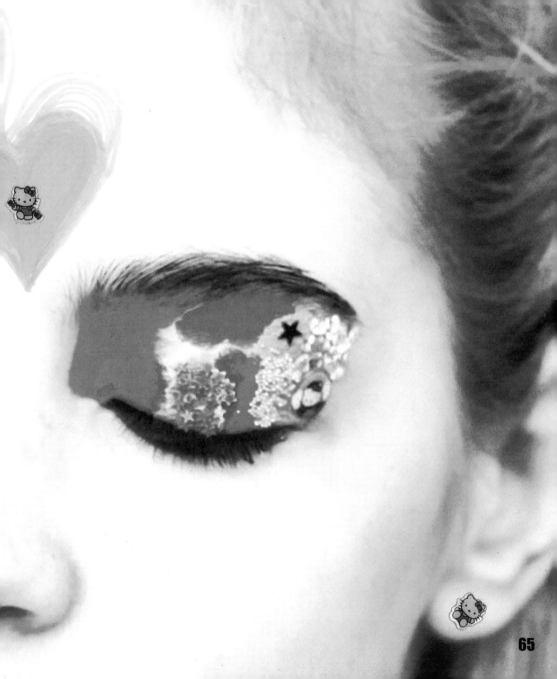

BRUSHES/TOOLS

If you're gonna go pro and compete with fifty billion make-up artists in this world, you're gonna have to invest in some fancy brushes. You might be surprised at the price of your new tools so I'm going to warn you now: expect to spend a reasonable amount on the essential members of your new brush family.

Once you've bought your key pieces from the more expensive stores, you can always add to your collection with a few online bargains. You'll need to build a decent selection to create a range of different make-up looks.

CROWN BRUSHES
make the best tools by far. They're amazing professional brushes at a good price. Go here to buy: **crownbrush.co.uk/ crownbrush.com/crownbrush.com.au**

ELF STUDIO
make decent brushes at astonishingly cheap prices. Go here and see for yourself: **eyeslipsface.co.uk/eyeslipsface.com/ elfcosmetics.com.au**

As a professional make-up artist, I personally recommend the **MAC Short Duo Fibre** Brush as officially, **IMO the BEST FOUNDATION BRUSH EVER.**

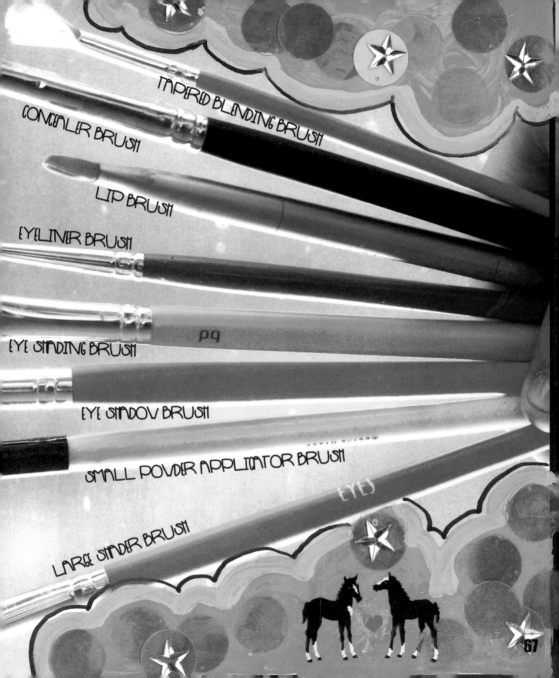

TAPERED BLENDING BRUSH

CONCEALER BRUSH

LIP BRUSH

EYELINER BRUSH

EYE SHADING BRUSH

pg

EYE SHADOW BRUSH

SMALL POWDER APPLICATOR BRUSH

EYES

LARGE SHADER BRUSH

67

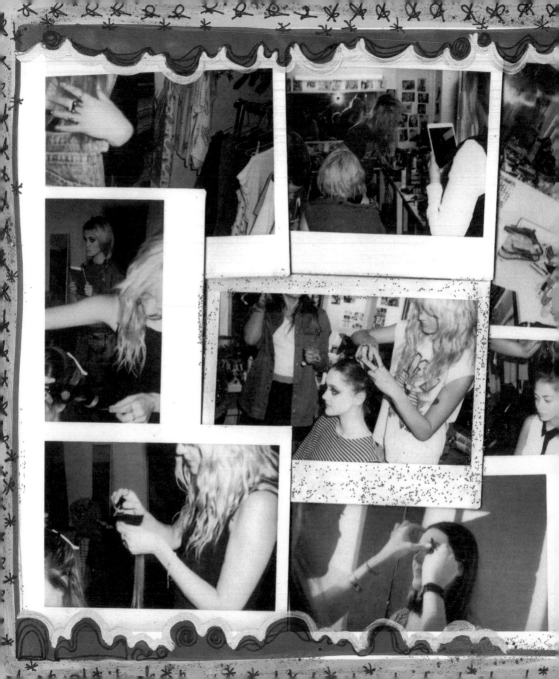

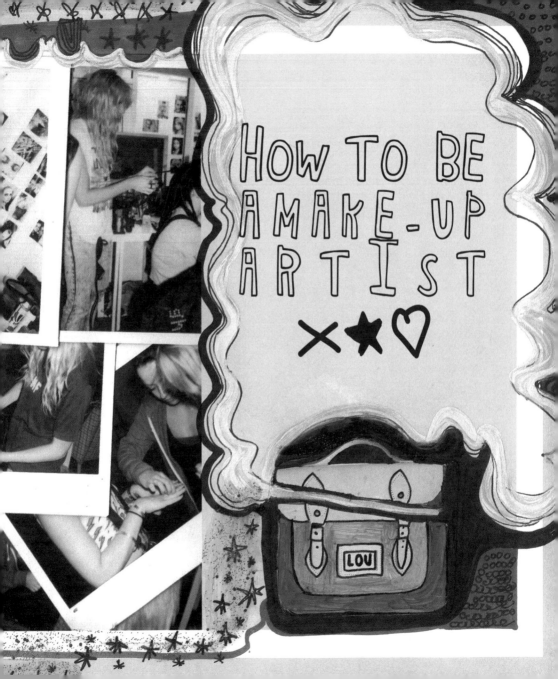

How to be a MAKE-UP ARTIST

X ★ ♡

LOU

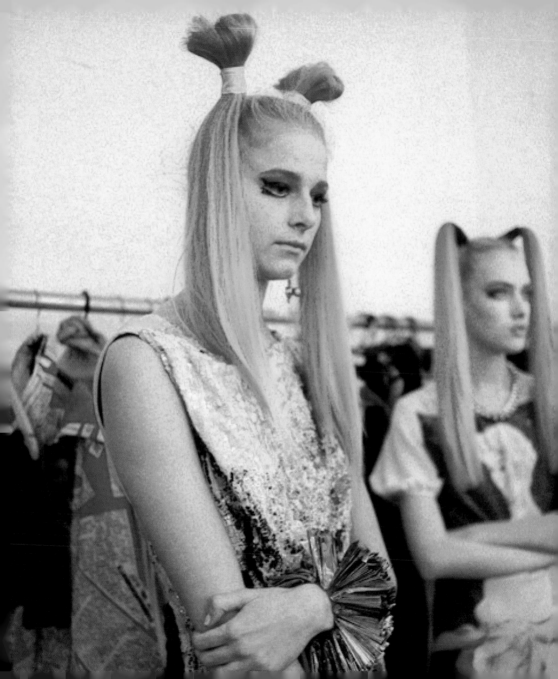

GETTING STARTED

If you ever speak to a hair or make-up artist you'll realise that EVERYONE got started in a different way. I believe there's no right or wrong way. There's also no 'fast track' to realising your dream. You need to work hard, have a good attitude and be in it for the long haul. Getting ANY job that is rewarding and fun takes time: long days, low pay and probably an unpleasant boss or two somewhere along the way. But if you keep practising, learning and improving, and you're the nicest person in the room at all times, then one day you'll earn good money and be super-happy!

One of the first ways to get started is to focus on the right subjects at school. If you're naturally creative and good at art then that's a great place to start,m and a key subject to concentrate on. Part of being in the industry is also about managing and marketing yourself. Subjects like business studies, cosmetology, media studies, fashion, marketing and I.T are all good courses to take if your school or college offer them.

Art schools in major fashion cities like London and New York offer specialized degrees in make-up. These are great if you're lucky enough to get on one. I went to the London College of Fashion and studied for three years, which gave me time to experiment and develop my practical ability. There are also many short courses available, which have very few entry requirements but tend to be really expensive. This route is good for those who might not have been successful in gaining a place on a degree, but it doesn't make you an expert any quicker! Treat it as the beginning of your training, learn the basics, then spend the next couple of years assisting, taking other courses and doing your own shoots. Short courses churn out hundreds of 'qualified' make-up artists every month and being in the same position as all these people isn't going to get you a paid job. You need to do more than everyone else, be the best, be the most productive, have five times the work experience everyone else has had AND take every opportunity that comes your way.

STUDYING

ASSISTING

Assisting established hair and make-up artists is the most important path to success in this industry. You may feel like you're not doing much make-up or hair and you're not earning any money, but it's the most effective way to start gathering your own clients when you're ready. I have had two amazing assistants in the last ten years and they both now work more than me and began to do so quickly! I have also had a lot more bad assistants who didn't do what it takes, worked the bare minimum and constantly asked for things. That approach doesn't work. You can't learn about an industry and how to behave without experience. If you're lucky enough to get an opportunity to assist someone, my advice is to be humble and make yourself indispensable to them!

POINTERS

1. Call your lead before the job and ask if there's anything they need you to do to prepare (they may need you to buy things for the kit, prepare references, clean etc.). Even if you have to head around late the night before to do it – offer!

2. Always make sure you set off to arrive at least fifteen minutes earlier than they tell you. NEVER be late. Never, ever!

3. During or after set-up, offer to get drinks and food for your lead. Always be considerate and try to make their day as nice and easy as possible. This would make me re-book you and fight for a fee for you if nothing else!

4. If you have no direction and are not doing much, also offer the client a drink. Your lead will be happy that you're keeping the client happy too!

5. When at a loose end… CLEAN! There is always cleaning and tidying to be done. If the brushes are clean and the table is tidy, have a look at the kit bags and see if there's any organising you can do to make things neater in there.

6. Make lists! Ask your lead if there's anything they are low on and offer to nip out to get anything needed.

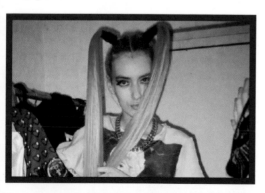

POINTERS

7. DON'T EVER take pictures on your phone and definitely don't ever put them online! It's so unprofessional and will lead to you being removed from the shoot immediately. DO talk to your lead about their own social networking and what they need help with on the day. A lot of big hairdressers and make-up artists in fashion have product sponsors and like to Tweet pics of them working on models throughout the day from their accounts. Being hot on this can make you invaluable to someone as they quite often don't have the time to do it.

8. Finish up properly and don't ask what time you're allowed to leave! See it through in an upbeat way and be as efficient as possible, by getting everything sorted for the lead artist. Offer to organise travel and don't bug them about your own.

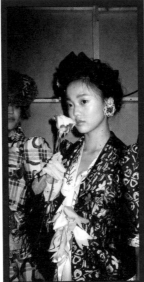

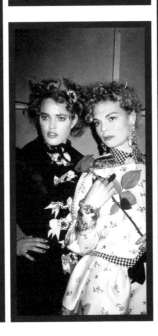

BECOME A JUNIOR

If hair is your main focus then you need to learn how to do hair. Even if make-up is your interest, if you wanna do celebrity work, or work with men, or simply work every day, then you need to know both! So simply getting a junior job in a salon could be more beneficial to you than a course, whilst earning you money rather than costing you. Hair is technical, there is a lot to learn and you can't learn enough. There is always more you can pick up so getting started early is the best thing to do. Once you have a bit of experience there are salons in bigger cities that have a focus on their hairdressers working in the session industry, like during fashion week or on TV shows. Getting a job doing this and being a star pupil can be one of the best routes to becoming your own artist.

73

If you want to be your own artist you need an identity and you need to be interesting. There are so many platforms to market yourself on nowadays and you need to utilise them. Pictures, articles, demos and product reviews are just a few simple things you can blog to get going. Just try adding some personality!

BLOGGING

If you want to focus on becoming a make-up artist then you might find getting a job on a make-up counter more beneficial than a course – and you get paid! The best way to learn make-up is to PRACTICE, PRACTICE, PRACTICE. And on a counter you'll do just that. Making up normal faces all day with the best products is a really good way to become very good at make-up.

WORKING ON A COUNTER

You'll actually get a lot more from doing this than any course and like the salons, you can work your way up in this sector and find yourself working for a top brand that supplies artists for fashion week.

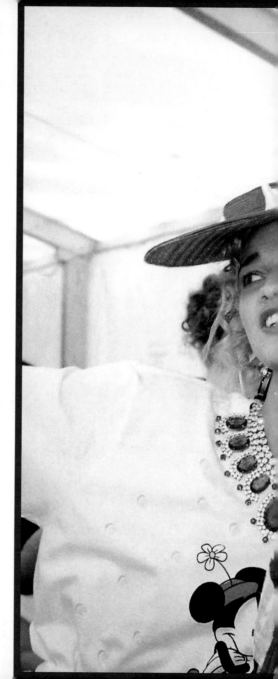

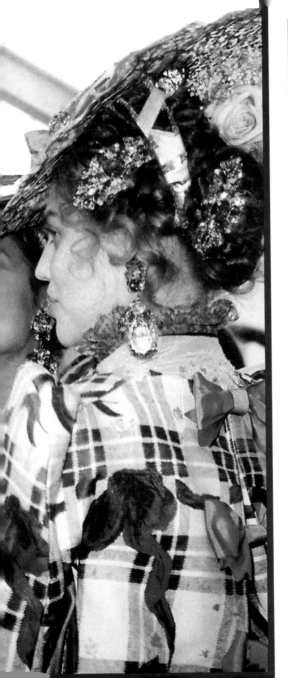

LOCATION LOCATION LOCATION

If you wanna work in the movies or at fashion week then you're no good living somewhere where they don't shoot any movies or have any fashion shows. Think realistically about how much you want to do this and decide if it's worth moving, because you won't work unless you live where there's an industry. If you're too young and penniless to move for a few years the best thing to do is work as a hairdresser and train in as many things as you can, save your money and make the move later. Both of my favourite assistants who work with huge celebrities now used to work in small salons out of the city and are simply very good at hair so got working very quickly in London.

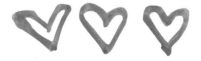

FASHION // MUSIC // FILM & TV

Once you have decided you want to do hair and make-up, you need to decide whether music and fashion or film and TV is for you. These two sides of the industry are very different and require specialised training. Music and fashion are very much about trends, beauty and personality. You need to be knowledgable and creative and assist and shoot as much as possible. Film and TV are very different. You need to train to use prosthetic make-up and

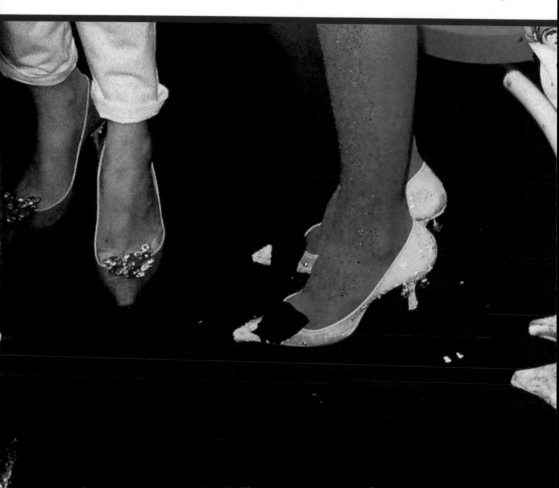

learn how to create effects. A lot of people start working in theatres and go from there, or get on a course to learn. If you're particularly good at life drawing or sculpture in art then this is more for you. The main piece of advice I can give to anyone wanting to get into the industry is to have a good, hard-working attitude and be willing to learn everything properly. If you're always nice, and good at your job, then people will want you back.

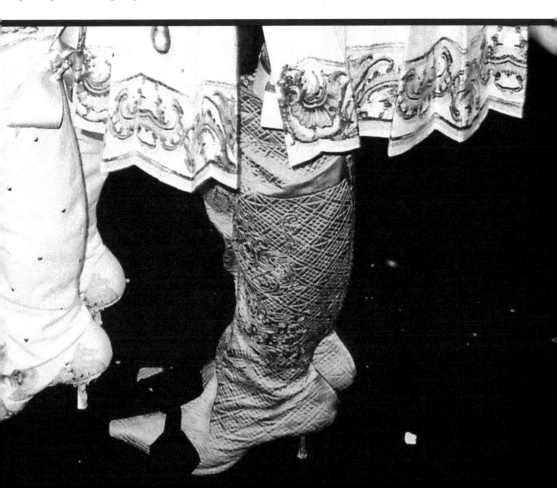

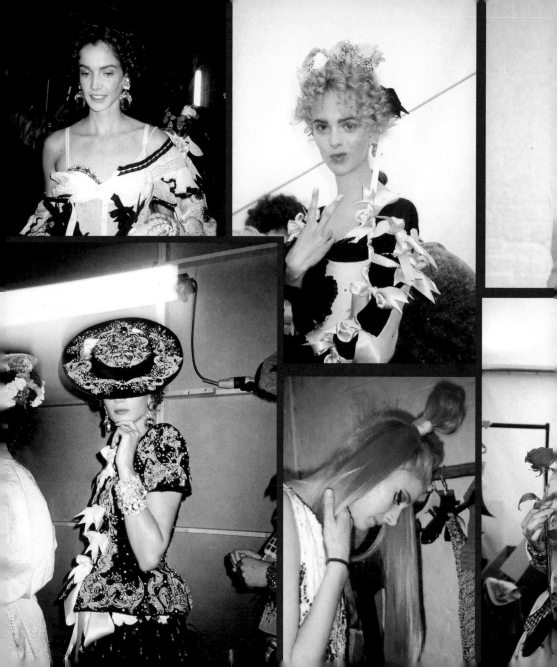

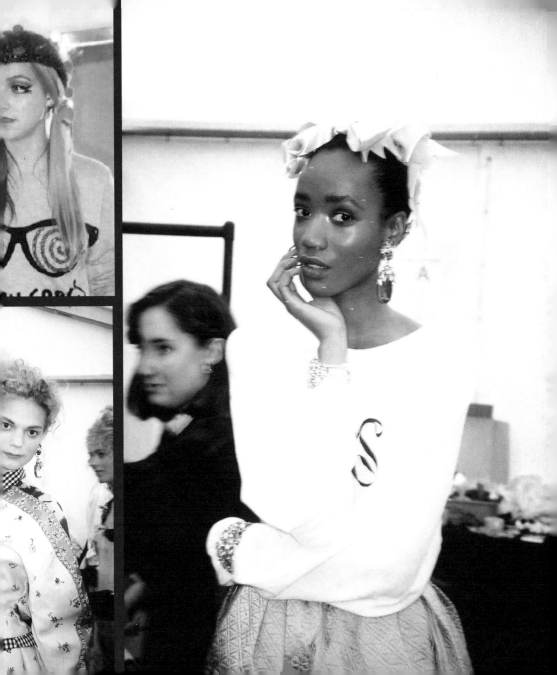

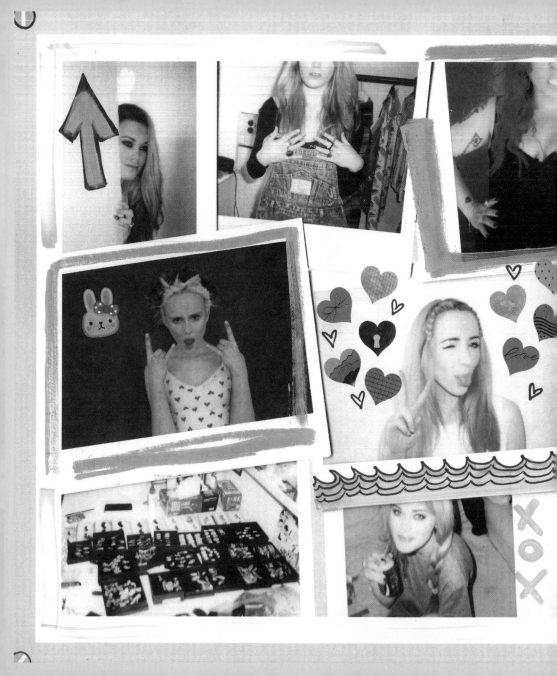

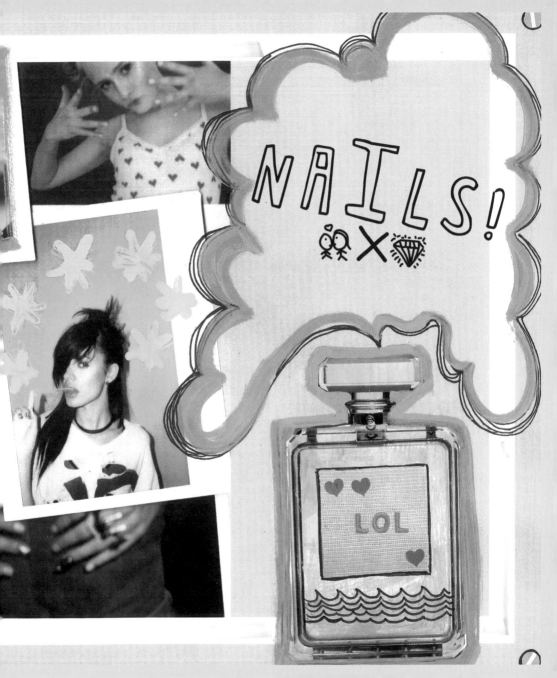

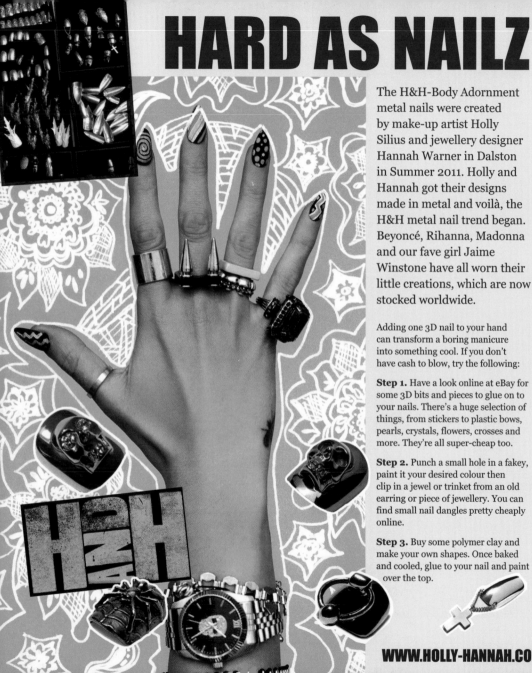

HARD AS NAILZ

The H&H-Body Adornment metal nails were created by make-up artist Holly Silius and jewellery designer Hannah Warner in Dalston in Summer 2011. Holly and Hannah got their designs made in metal and voilà, the H&H metal nail trend began. Beyoncé, Rihanna, Madonna and our fave girl Jaime Winstone have all worn their little creations, which are now stocked worldwide.

Adding one 3D nail to your hand can transform a boring manicure into something cool. If you don't have cash to blow, try the following:

Step 1. Have a look online at eBay for some 3D bits and pieces to glue on to your nails. There's a huge selection of things, from stickers to plastic bows, pearls, crystals, flowers, crosses and more. They're all super-cheap too.

Step 2. Punch a small hole in a fakey, paint it your desired colour then clip in a jewel or trinket from an old earring or piece of jewellery. You can find small nail dangles pretty cheaply online.

Step 3. Buy some polymer clay and make your own shapes. Once baked and cooled, glue to your nail and paint over the top.

WWW.HOLLY-HANNAH.COM

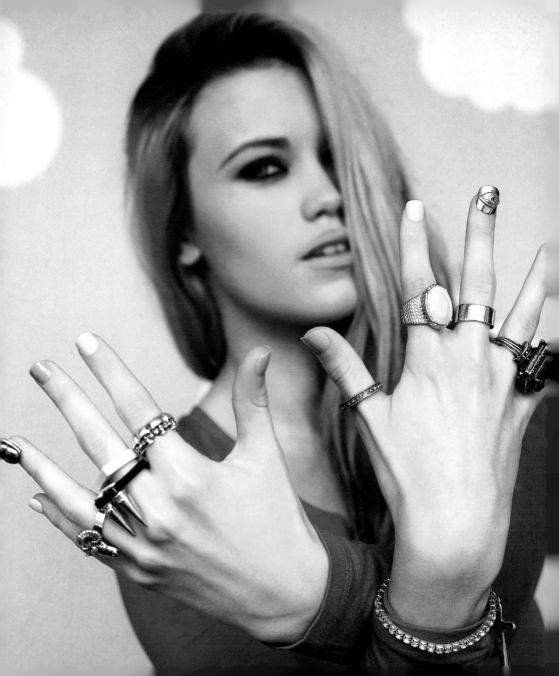

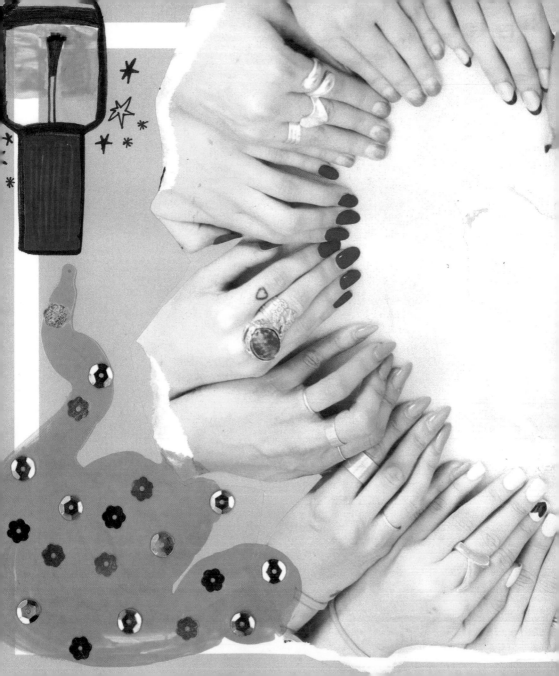

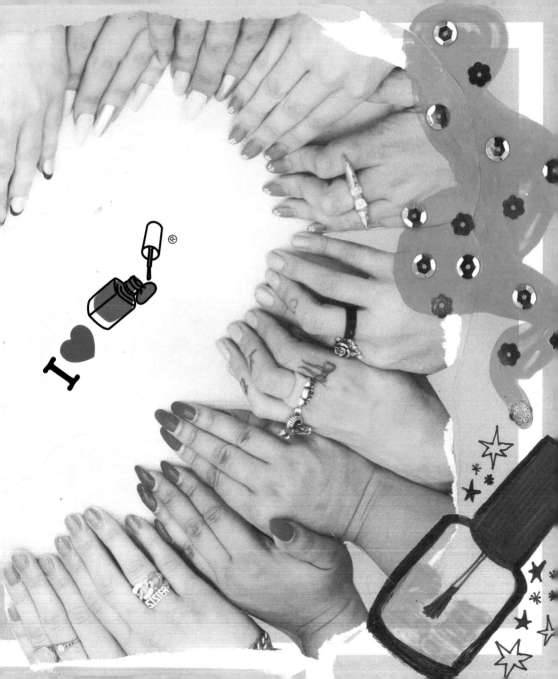

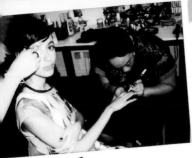

AMA

NAIL ARTIST: AMA QUASHIE

BASE, TOP COAT & CUTICLE OIL

The holy trinity of a long-lasting manicure, don't even think about painting your nails without these three. Base coat protects your nail bed along with the top coat, which sandwiches the colour in. Cuticle oil gives your nails a professional finish while keeping your cuticles moisturised. My three absolute must-haves are: *Bonder Rubberized Basecoat by Orly*, *Seche Vite Top Coat* and lastly *Essie's Apricot Cuticle Oil*.

Superstar nail guru Ama Quashie works as a nail artist in the fashion industry doing funky nails on fashion shoots and music videos ... and we've got all her nail secrets for you! :)

QUICK DRY

When you're in a rush and need your nails to dry that little bit faster, forget those sprays that you've probably been subjected to in your local nail shop. Go get yourself *Revlon's Liquid Quick Dry*. Lightly brush it over your nails around five minutes after you've top-coated and voilà!

FAKEYS

Whether it's to add a little length and glamour for a special occasion or just because you don't want acrylics, press-on nails are an amazingly quick, effective and cheap alternative. *Kiss* have a great full cover nails in a range of shapes, and while you're there, pick yourself up some nail tabs to stick them on with.

5 KIT ESSENTIALS

*CLEAN-UP BRUSH

For cleaning up the edges of your manicure, nail supply shops will stock them. Alternatively you can use a thin make-up brush. My favourite is *Revlon's Concealer Brush*.

NAIL VARNISH THINNER

Don't listen to the old wives tale and use nail varnish remover to revive/thin down your polish. Over time it will only ruin the remaining polish by breaking down its chemical structure. Invest in actual thinner – yes it does exist and my kit isn't complete without one. *OPI's Nail Lacquer Thinner* is amazing!

FOLLOW @NAILSBYAMA

nailsbyama.tumblr.com

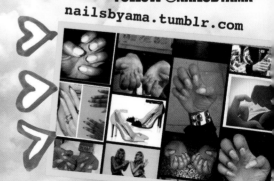

DIY TIPS:

LAYERS

A mistake that a lot of people make is to do a complete design on one nail, then move onto the next. All this usually does is make the colours bleed into one another and makes the design a messy. The key is to break down your design into layers – paint each layer onto all ten fingers before moving onto the next then go back to the first finger again and do it until your nail art is finished. This gives the varnish time to dry between layers.

NAIL ON A NAIL

One of the best pieces of advice I was ever given when I started doing nails was to paint the shape of a nail onto your nail, rather than trying to fill it. Paint all the way to the top of the cuticle, place your brush at the top-middle of your nail as close to the cuticle as you can get without actually letting the paint touch it. Then make a stroke to the left following the line of your nail bed, repeat on the right-hand side and then finish off by carefully painting over the free edge. The key is to paint thinly and evenly – too much polish in one coat will only lengthen how long it takes for your nails to dry.

' SIMPLICITY: IN MY OPINION, NAIL ART DOESN'T ALWAYS HAVE TO BE EVERYTHING ALL AT ONCE JUST FOR THE SAKE OF IT – THE SIMPLEST OF DESIGNS CAN MAKE JUST AS MUCH IMPACT. '

*To give your manicure a professional edge, all good manicurists use a little brush to clean the cuticle line and edges of any imperfetions. Simply dab the brush into some acetone/nail varnish remover and slide the brush along the perimeter of your nail.

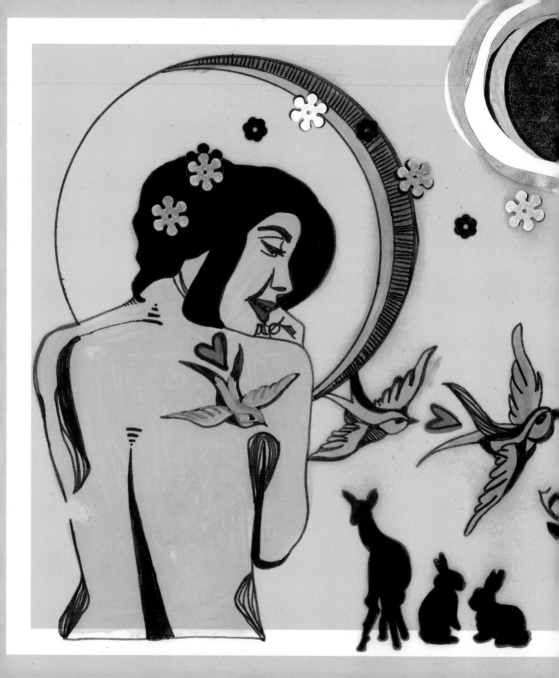

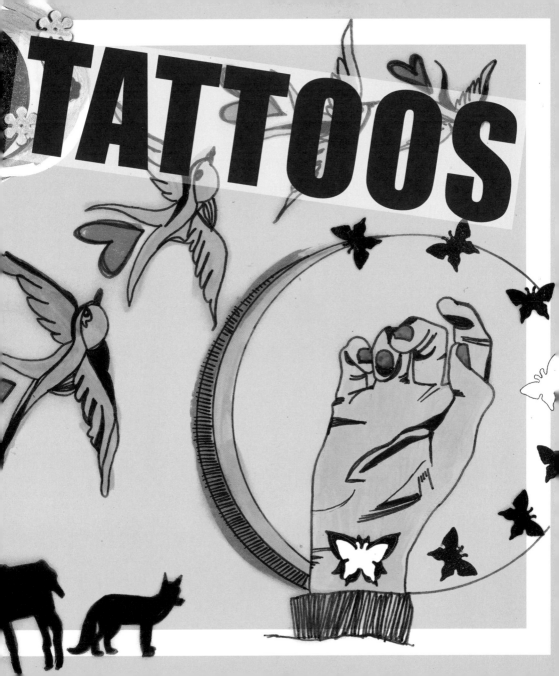

TATTOOS

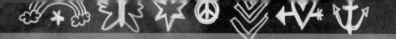

TATTOO BABE: ELLIE MAY, LONDON

How did you decide what tattoos to have and why?

I've never actually known what I wanted to have tattooed until about ten minutes before the artist is about to stick the needle in! It was always more about the artist themselves and having a piece of their work on my skin. With my roses, I was in love with an artist called Amanda Toy and I finally managed to get a spot when she was in London. She came up with the idea, drew it, and it just fit perfectly.

Do you have any regrets?

The first tattoo I had was stupid and not for the right reasons. I went and got it up the inside of my forearm too, which was really dumb! Now I have three shooting stars on my arm – completely regret that. But I think regret is a good thing! You learn from your mistakes (blah, blah, blah!) and I can always get it covered up.

When will you stop getting tattooed?

I don't think I'll ever stop. Apart from my first, I've only ever got tattoos for myself and as long as I have an interest in the art behind it, I'll keep on getting tattooed.

How do your tattoos affect your everyday life?

They haven't ever really affected me. I've never been asked to cover them up for a job and when I first got into tattoos I decided I'd never want to work for anyone who would think ink on my skin would affect my work. Tattoos still have stigma with the older generation and people think it's OK sometimes to blatantly voice their disgust out loud. I always find the best way to deal with this is to make it clear you would never be so openly rude about something they were wearing or the way they've done their hair. The best way to change people's minds is not to conform to stereotypes, so don't be rude or disrespectful!

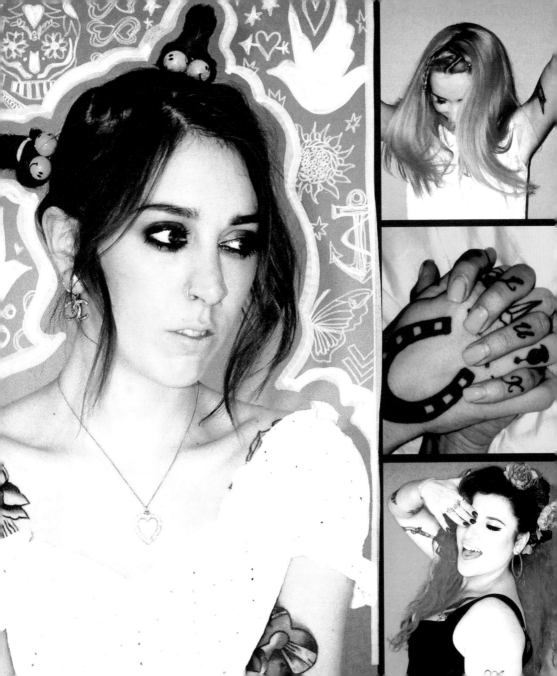

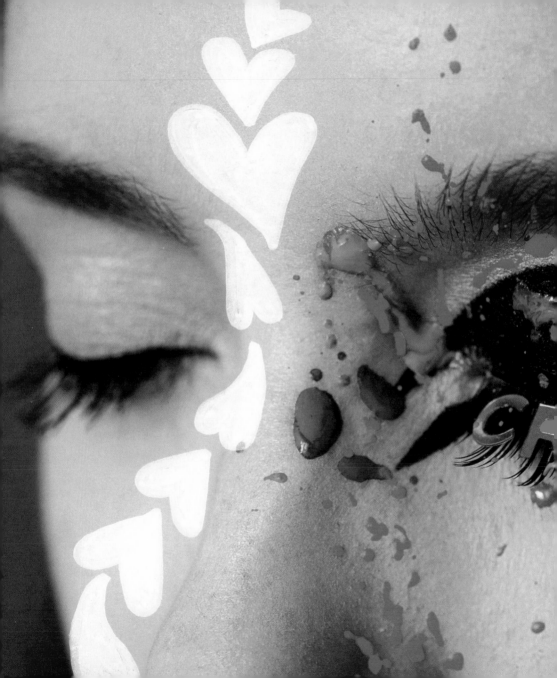

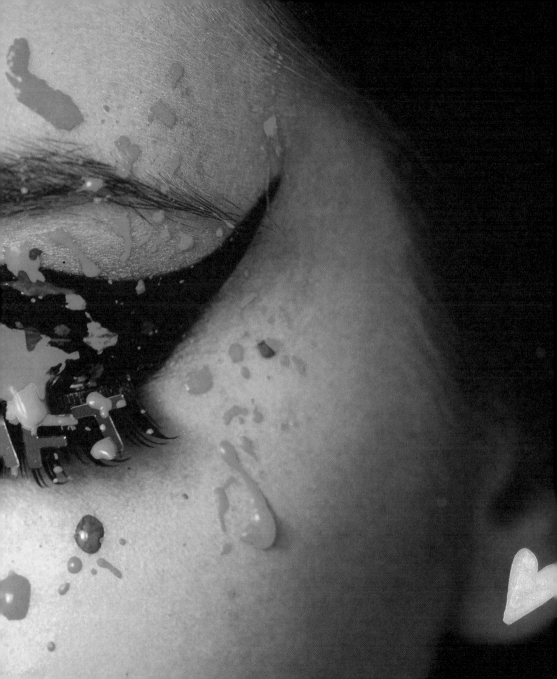

THANK YOUS

THANK you to Krystal, my amazing agent for pretty much doing EVERYTHING on this book while I've been away all year – and I'm sorry my days off to shoot this were on your weekend! Also to Eve, who has laid out the whole thing and made it look exactly how I wanted without even having to ask. Thanks Faran for illustrating everything sooooo beautifully and taking us partying in New York – sorry we made you go in Hogs and Heffers, not v cool. Thank you to my amazing assistants Kara, Polly and Lottie and Justin Borbely and Masha Mel for shooting all the images. Thanks to Ama and Josie for all the super nails and Hannah and Brad for all the amazing hair colour. Thank yooooou Kahlani twins for being so cute and cool and good at what you both do. I hope we work together forever I think you're amazing. Thanks Rebecca Wilson for invaluable advice and Gemma for proofreading – you should be a teacher :) and all the gorgeous models that came along and let me change their hair colour! Thanks Sam for being a 'stylist' for the day and Holly for coming and bringing some sparkles! Thanks Fudge Urban for such huge support (and Jules from St Tropez for your amazing super tans and tips) and last but not least Hardie Grant for publishing me!

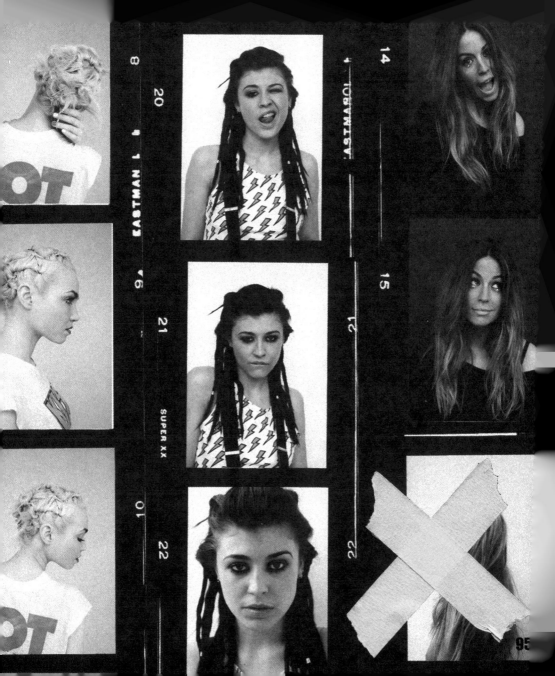

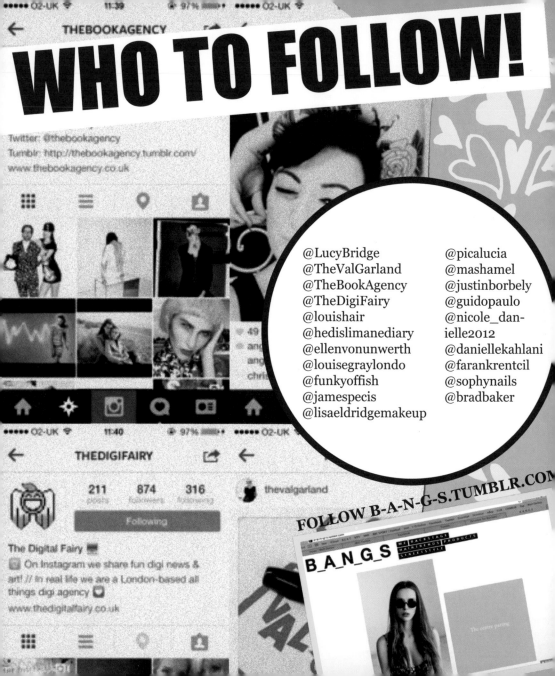

WHO TO FOLLOW!

Twitter: @thebookagency
Tumblr: http://thebookagency.tumblr.com/
www.thebookagency.co.uk

@LucyBridge
@TheValGarland
@TheBookAgency
@TheDigiFairy
@louishair
@hedislimanediary
@ellenvonunwerth
@louisegraylondo
@funkyoffish
@jamespecis
@lisaeldridgemakeup

@picalucia
@mashamel
@justinborbely
@guidopaulo
@nicole_dan-
ielle2012
@daniellekahlani
@farankrentcil
@sophynails
@bradbaker

THEDIGIFAIRY

| 211 posts | 874 followers | 316 following |

Following

thevalgarland

The Digital Fairy
On Instagram we share fun digi news & art! // In real life we are a London-based all things digi agency
www.thedigitalfairy.co.uk

FOLLOW B-A-N-G-S.TUMBLR.COM

B_A_N_G_S

The centre parting

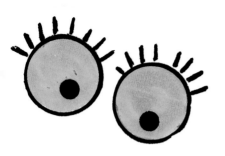

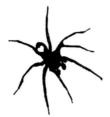

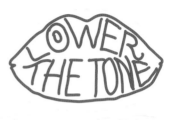

LOWER THE TONE

TARANTULA LASHES

DRAINBOW

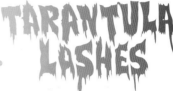

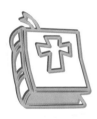

THE CRAFT

TARANTULA LASHES

BROWSCARA

LOL PERFUME

SUPER BASE

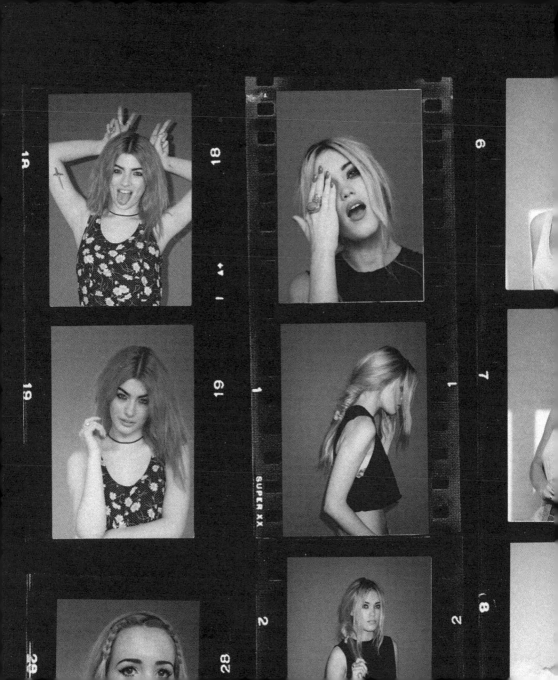